BODY TRANSFORMATION: GET LEAN OR BULK UP

BY

PAUL NAM

This information in this book is a guideline for reference. Before starting any diet or fitness program, consult your doctor, a dietitian or certified nutritionist. Any use of this information provided is at the user's risk.

For more works by this author, please visit:

www.pursefitness.com

www.theworkoutloft.com

https://payhip.com/wy2kool

https://theworkoutloft.com/online-training-programs

OTHER BOOKS BY THE AUTHOR

FIT TO FAT IN 8 WEEKS

SCRAWNY TO BRAWNY IN 8 WEEKS

NUTRITION 101: BUILDING THE FOUNDATION

IT'S ALL ABOUT YOUR HEALTH: FOOD RECIPES

THE BOOK OF CHOICES: THE LIVES OF 2 ATHLETES

IMMUNE SYSTEM 8: BOOST YOUR IMMUNE SYSTEM NATURALLY

DUMBBELL TRAINING: FOR MEN AND WOMEN

BODYBUILDING AND STEROIDS: MY PERSONAL STORY

DUMBBELL AND CORE(ABS) TRAINING : FOR MEN AND WOMEN

BEGINNER'S GUIDE TO DIET AND TRAINING

LEARN HOW TO STRETCH: FOR BETTER MOVEMENT AND HEALTH

FUSION FITNESS: NUTRITION AND WEIGHT LOSS COMBINED

THE ULTIMATE GUIDE TO CORE(ABS) TRAINING: NO MORE LOW BACK PAIN

TABLE OF CONTENTS

_____

INTRODUCTION

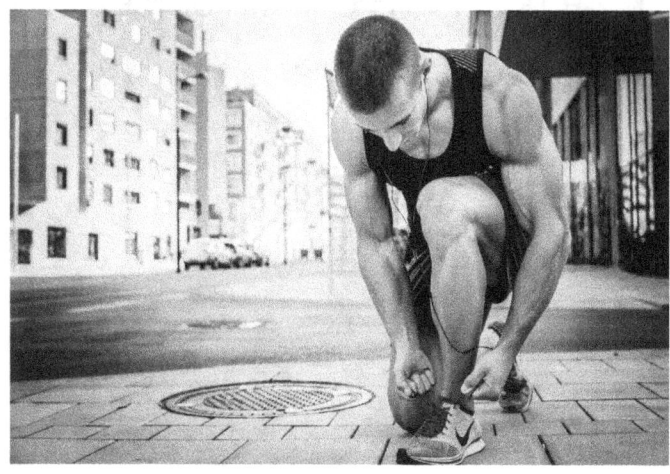

What does it take to get fit? That is a question most people have when they want to get into shape. Whether you want to gain muscle mass or lose bodyfat, both require work.

Welcome to Body Transformation: Get Lean Or Bulk Up. You have the choice either to get lean or bulk up and gain some serious muscle. The best way to build a physique is to bulk up first, then cut down. This is the process I would follow before my bodybuilding shows. The end result would be a physique that would turn heads at the beach. There is a process to follow and I have layed that out in this book. Good luck and train hard but smart!

SECTION A - LOSE FAT AND GET RIPPED

THE MAJOR NUTRIENTS

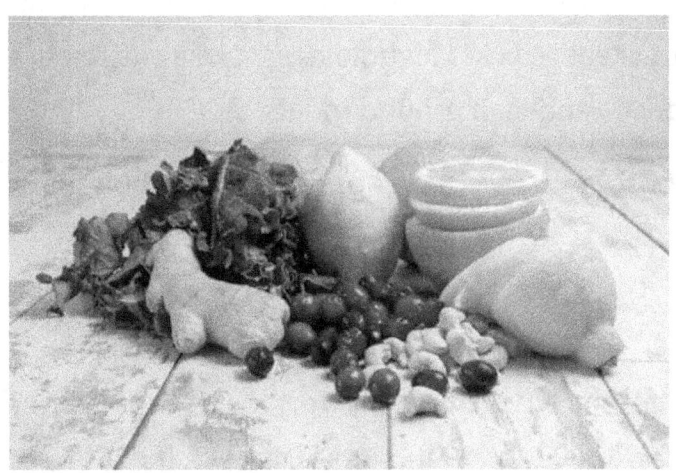

Here is an interesting fact.

Nutrients are needed by your body to provide structure, regulate your metabolism, and supply energy.

Protein is important for providing the structure of your muscles. Many vitamins help to regulate the hundreds of chemical reactions that happen in your body, and fats provide an important source of energy to power most of your body's activities.

This chapter will teach you briefly about the different classes of nutrients.

PROTEINS

Protein is found in many foods, such as meats, legumes, and some cereal products. The proteins that are in your body have many roles, including being an energy source. They are also a major structural material in many parts of your body, such as muscle, bone, and skin. Proteins allow us to move, works with the immune system to keep us healthy, and regulates many chemical reactions needed for life.

The best sources are steak, chicken, whole eggs, turkey, fish, pork, beans, protein powder, dairy products, and lean ground meats.

If you're vegan, choose tofu, seeds, quinoa, beans, and non- dairy protein powders.

CARBOHYDRATES

There are many different types of carbohydrates as those found in foods like rice and pasta, verses foods like fruits and desserts. The most important carbohydrate is glucose because our cells use glucose as their primary source of energy. Other than tasting good, carbohydrates are used for other purposes as well. Some are needed to make the DNA that is inside of your cells. Certain carbohydrates like dietary fiber helps to maintain the health of your digestive system. Like proteins, carbohydrates are also important structural components in the membranes that surround the cells in your body.

The best sources of carbohydrates should come from whole grains, fruits, and vegetables. Man-made carbohydrates, like pasta, should be secondary and it's best to limit or eliminate refined sugars, such as candy.

Now onto the next, fats.

FATS

Fats are found in a variety of oils, foods, and in the human body. They provide energy to the body, are important for the structure of cell membranes, and are needed for the development of your nervous and reproductive system.

Just remember one rule, eat more omega 3 than omega 6 fatty acids.

The best sources of fats come from fatty fish, omega 3, flax seed oil, nuts, seeds, extra virgin olive oil, avocados, and cheese.

WATER

Did you know water is made up of oxygen and hydrogen atoms?

Yawn, not a fun fact at all.

Water makes up about 60% of your total body weight so it is important to stay hydrated. The functions are very important as it helps to transport nutrients, gases, and waste products. Water also helps to regulate your body temperature and protects your internal organs from damage.

The suggested guideline for water intake for adult females is 10-11 cups of water daily from both drinks and food. Men should have 13-14 cups of water from drinks and food.

VITAMINS

Vitamins are found in most foods but are abundant in fruits, vegetables, and grains. Your body needs vitamins to regulate chemical reactions and to promote growth and development. Some vitamins are called antioxidants, which help to protect your body from toxic compounds such as air pollution.

Vitamins are classified as either water or fat soluble. The fat soluble vitamins are A,D,E,K, and the water soluble vitamins are B, and C.

The best sources for vitamins are raw fruits, raw vegetables, grains, meats, and dairy products.

MINERALS

Some minerals such as Iron, selenium, and sodium are found in the earth. Minerals are called inorganic substance, which the exception of water. Most minerals are essential nutrients, each serving it's own purpose. An example would be sodium, which helps to regulate water balance in your body. Minerals are not used as an energy source but help with energy producing- reactions.

All foods contain minerals so if you eat a balanced diet of carbohydrates, fats, and protein, there should be no deficiencies.

UNDERSTANDING THE ENERGY EQUATION

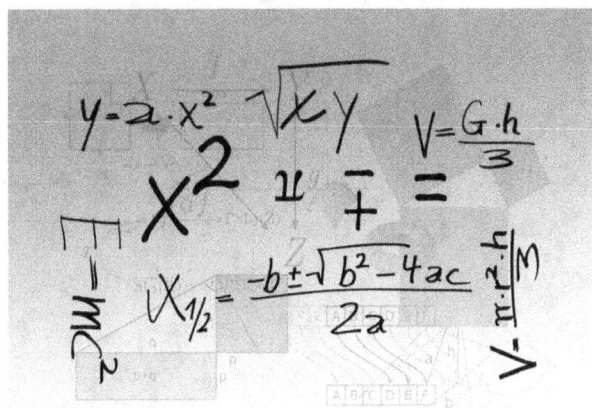

What is energy? Energy is defined as the capacity or power to do work, such as moving an object by the use of force. Understanding the energy equation will help you shed fat and gain muscle faster.

To do physical activity you need energy, which comes from the foods we eat. Throughout this chapter, we will be going through energy balance, how it affects body weight, and energy expenditure.

Energy balance is a state in which energy intake equals the energy burned. An example would be if a person were to eat 2000 calories a day and then burn 2000 calories that same day. Energy imbalances happen when the amount of energy consumed does not equal the amount of energy used.

Energy imbalances result in a positive or negative energy imbalance. Positive energy imbalance is a state where energy intake is greater than the energy expenditure. An example of a positive energy imbalance would be a person eating 3000 calories and sitting down all day and watching television burning only 1200 calories. Negative energy balance is when energy intake is less that the energy expenditure. An example of negative energy balance is when a person eats 1000 calories and exercises for 3 hours and walks around all day burning 1100 calories.

Understanding energy intake and expenditure is one way to keep the body weight stable. When energy intake equals energy expenditure, the body weight becomes stable. In a state of positive energy balance, the body weight increases. When energy intake is in a negative balance, the body weight decreases.

During positive energy balance a person either gains body fat or muscle mass and this depends of what type of activity they are engaging in. Gaining body weight is considered healthy during growth periods during infancy, childhood, and pregnancy.

What is not considered healthy is when a person is in a positive energy balance from being inactive and gains excessive body fat.

Why do people eat food other than for survival and for enjoyment? Hunger and satiety are somewhat complex physiological states that influence the amount of food a person eats. Satiety is a state in which hunger is satisfied and a person feels that they had enough to eat. Hunger is defined as the physiological drive to consume food. Both hunger and satiety are influenced by factors such as gastric (stomach) stretching, circulation nutrient level, and gastrointestinal hormones.

What is a food craving?

A food craving is a very strong desire for a particular food and is different from hunger. Simply put, a food craving is satisfied when the person eats that desired food. Women seem to experience more food cravings then men do. This could be due to the hormonal changes during their menstrual cycles.

During pregnancy, the fluctuations of hormones may cause some women to crave certain foods. Following an over-restrictive diet could also cause food cravings. When I used to diet for bodybuilding competitions, I would restrict sugars, salt, carbs, and certain kinds of fats for 10 weeks. After 2-3 weeks of eating a restrictive diet I would crave certain foods like burgers and chocolate bars. To keep on track and to defeat these food cravings I would allow myself a cheat meal once a week. This would allow me to look forward to that certain day where I would be able to eat whatever I was craving. This is an effective way to stay on track with your eating guidelines if your goal is to lose body fat. Getting enough sleep, exercising regularly, eating a wide variety of healthy foods are other factors to help these food cravings.

We have gone over energy in and energy out, however energy intake is only half of the energy balance equation.

The other half is called energy expenditure. The components that make up energy expenditure are basal metabolism, physical activity, and the thermic effect of food. The thermic effect of food is the energy required to process food and is roughly 10% of total energy expenditure (TEE). Physical energy is the energy required for body movement and is about 15% to 30% of TEE. Basal metabolism is the energy required for basic life function and is roughly 50% to 70% of TEE.

The basal metabolism is the biggest factor of all 3, so the best way to increase your metabolism is building your muscle mass through resistance training. Muscle mass burns more calories at rest than fat mass.

Most health practitioners know what BMR is and use it to assess people. Basal metabolic rate is the energy used for basal metabolism, which is expressed as kcal per hour. In simple terms, BMR is the amount of calories a person burns at rest.

BMR accounts for 50-70% of TEE and is measured in the morning, during a fasted state, after 8 hours of sleep, and in a temperature controlled room.

Trying to figure out a person's BMR can be a challenge since it requires so many conditions to gather an accurate reading, clinicians often measure resting metabolic rate instead (RMR). RMR is around 10% higher than BMR. When resting metabolism is used over a 24-hour period, it is called resting energy expenditure (REE).

To figure out a person's REE, clinicians use a formula called the Harris Benedict equation, as shown below. If you don't want to calculate it manually, you can always Google the Harris Benedict equation and punch in the numbers.

Males: REE = 66.5 + [13.8 x weight (kg)] + [5 x height (cm)] - [6.8 x age (y)]

Females: REE = 655.1 + [9.6 x weight (kg)] + [1.8 x height (cm)] - [4.7 x age (y)]

As we age, our ability to burn the same amount of calories at rest declines about 2- 5% every 10 years. Add menopause for females, and male pattern baldness to the mix and it doesn't sound like too much fun at all. People with more muscle mass usually have a higher BMR than people with more fat mass. This is because muscle has greater metabolic activity than fat tissue.

As we age, our muscle mass also decreases. These reasons and more are why a person should always include resistance training in their training program.

One of the most interesting factors that can affect a person's BMR is food restriction or extreme dieting. When a person restricts calories over a period of time, they will lose both body fat and muscle.

Another thing that can happen is your BMR slowing down in response to a negative energy balance. This is why some people hit a plateau when dieting over a long period of time.

Physical activity is the second largest part of the total energy expenditure equation and makes up 15-30% of the total equation.

Activities like resistance training, biking, swimming, and walking burn more calories than walking.

Body mass and size also influence energy expended during physical activities. Smaller people have less body mass than a larger person so they would naturally burn fewer calories when doing the same exercise such as running.

Lastly, is the thermic effect of food (TEF). TEF is defined as energy expended for the digestion and absorption of nutrients. Some foods like steak require more energy to break down than others.

High fat foods have the lowest TEF while protein has highest TEF. This does not mean to cut out all high fat food and eat all protein and expect to burn more calories.

Thermic effect of food is only 5 to 10% of the total energy equation. All 3 play an important role together in the quest to burn body fat or build muscle.

EATING FOR FAT LOSS

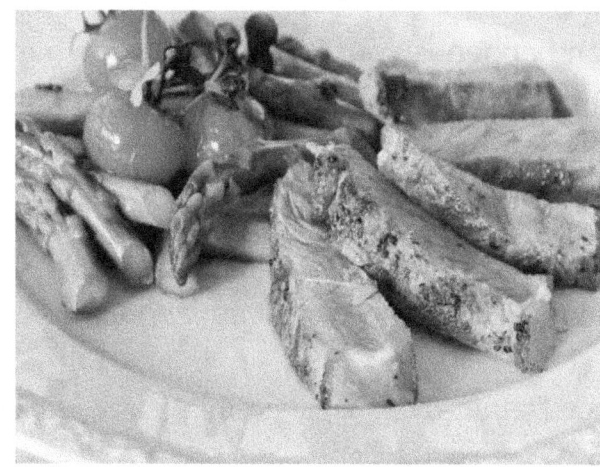

Your stomach starts to growl and you start to think about food.

Why do we need to eat?

Humans need to eat in order to have energy for every day movements. What happens when a person's every movement becomes limited because of a sedentary job or an injury? As we have learned earlier, if a person's energy intake is greater than their energy output, body fat tissue is formed.

Throughout this chapter, we'll be learning about adipose tissue, SCAT and VAT, eating habits that contribute to obesity, and eating for fat loss.

Adipose tissue is made up of lipid-filled cells called adipocytes, which contain a core of triglycerides. The number and size of adipocytes determine the mass of adipose in a person's body. If a person is in consistent positive energy balance, their adipocytes start to fill up with triglyceride. When that adipocyte if full, a new one is formed and the process continues. When a person loses body fat, the enlarged adipocyte shrinks back to normal size but the number of adipocytes remain the same. This is why when a person loses 20 lbs. from following a successful weight loss plan, they gain the weight back fast as soon as they go back to eating junk food and larger food portions.

Inside the human body, adipose tissue is found throughout the body. Visceral adipose tissue (VAT) is defined as tissue deposited between the internal organs and the abdominal area. Subcutaneous adipose tissue (SCAT) is adipose tissue that is found beneath the skin. VAT is considered more of a health risk than SCAT because the intra-abdominal fat is more likely to undergo lipolysis. Lipolysis is the breakdown of a triglyceride molecule into glycerol and fatty acids.

This may cause an increase in levels of LDL (bad) cholesterol, insulin, and a decrease in HDL (good) cholesterol. Other conditions such as high blood pressure, type 2 diabetes, and inflammation may become more prevalent due to having excessive intra-abdominal fat.

Overeating and inactivity are 2 main causes that contribute to obesity. We now know that being in a consistent positive energy balance can make a person gain adipose tissue. There are many societal and physiological factors that can influence the amount of food a person eats.

Two can dine for $8.99? Who could say no to such a deal? But what we don't all know is that this popular value meal can pack 1350 calories (for one person), which is more than half of the daily energy requirements. These types of fast foods are energy dense, inexpensive, readily available, and accepted as the cultural norm. Societal influence can affect the amount and what type of food people eat. We often see advertisements and commercials every day for these types of food. Studies have also shown that people tend to eat more if the serving size is larger. Do you think about portion size when you go to an all you can eat buffet? I try not go to all you can eat buffets as it usually ends in stomachache from excessive food consumption.

Obesity can also result from having poor self-esteem. Eating food can make a person feel good and some people eat to cope with stress. Obese individuals may experience depression and panic attacks more than people who are at a normal weight. A person's social network may also affect if they gain weight or not. If all of your friends eat fast food all the time and do not exercise, there is a good chance you will do the same.

Eating for fat loss can be one of the most challenging and confusing aspects, since there are so many so-called experts out there with different opinions on fat loss. After training over 1000 people and competing in over 20 bodybuilding shows, I have formulated my own recipe for success that requires some simple steps.

The first step is to figure out a person's BMR. A male who is 35 years old, 172 cm tall, weighs 165 lbs. has an BMR of 1706 kcal per day. So he would need at least 1706 kcal per day to maintain normal body functions. Next step is to figure out his caloric intake using a calorie counting app like MyFitnessPal or an online counting system. If he has a BMR of 1706 kcal per day and is ingesting over 2400 calories per day, he would be in a positive energy balance. In order to lose body fat, he would then have to exercise to burn off those extra calories.

Exercising can consist of cardiovascular or resistance workouts, or a combination of both. A combination of both is recommended as they both burn calories and work different areas.

Cardiovascular workouts are good for your heart, lungs, and VO2 max while resistance training is good for building muscle mass. As we have learned earlier, muscle mass burns more calories at rest. So, if he did 2 cardiovascular workouts and burned 300 calories at each session, then he completed 2 resistance-training workouts and burned 200 calories at each, the total calories burned would be 1000 calories for the week, putting him at 1400 (2400-1000) calories for the week. Remember, his BMR is 1706 kcal per day and this would put him in a negative energy balance (1706-1400= -306) where weight loss would occur. If he was to ingest 2800 calories a day and did not want to give up some junk food, I would suggest for him to do another workout to burn off some extra calories. Our bodies do not like extreme changes as it works to maintain homeostasis all the time.

There are 3 things you need to cut gradually back on which are sugars, carbohydrates, and certain fats. Sugars and carbohydrates both raise your insulin levels and this promotes fat storage. Fats are 9 calories per gram so cutting back will automatically lighten up a person's caloric intake. Just remember a simple rule, eat more omega 3 fats. Another rule I use is not to eat sugars or carbohydrates after 6 pm. When a person wakes up they burn carbohydrates as a fuel source because their glycogen levels are low but at night carbohydrates are stored for later use. If you are hungry at night eat a small portion of protein and vegetables or just protein by itself. Just make sure you don't eat a 12-ounce steak before you go to bed, as anything in excess will be turned into body fat.

Should I eat every 2 or 3 hours and how many meals should I eat in a day? Meal timing and portion size is a crucial component when it comes to burning fat. Some experts say 3 meals and day and 2 snacks. Others say 3 meals and 3 protein shakes a day. There is no perfect system to lose weight but what I usually recommend 3 meals and 1-2 snacks a day. If my clients are not reaching their REE and feel full I do not add extra calories to their meals as they may cause unwanted weight gain. I work with what they already eat and I just recommend healthier food choices. People who have kids and a full time job do not have time to eat 5-6 times a day. As for meal timing usually 2.5-3 hours between all meals or snacks will give the intestinal tract enough time to digest the food. The goal here is to figure out what works for you, as your metabolism is different from other people. What should I eat for a snack? I usually eat a 5 oz. protein serving with 1 cup of natural yogurt before I go to bed. This snack does not raise my insulin levels and keeps me full. Other good snack choices are natural cheese, Greek yogurt, small handful of nuts, vegetables and hummus, low carbohydrate protein bars, and slower-releasing protein powder. Another quick snack would be the meat leftovers from your supper. Next we will be going over portion sizes and two example meal plans for fat loss.

TWO EXAMPLE OF DIFFERENT EATING PLANS FOR FAT LOSS

EATING PLAN 1

This is an example of a fat loss diet for a male who is moderately active, can follow a low-carbohydrate diet, and would not have as much time to eat. He would eat 3 meals and 2 snacks a day.

A cheat meal with carbs would be allowed every 4th or 5th day. This is just an example diet as you can modify it to suit your needs.

If you have a hard time following a low-carb diet, then add 1 cup of carbs to the lunch. If you don't have much time for breakfast you can have snack 1 at 8:00 am and meal 1 at 3:00 pm. Please see next page.

Meal 1 8:00am	3 eggs(2 whole+1 white) with 1 slice cheese 1 cup grapes (fruit of your choice)
Meal 2 12:00pm	7-8oz pork with barbecue sauce 2 cup vegetables with Italian dressing
Snack 1 3:00pm	1 scoop whey or isolate powder 1 cup natural yogurt 1/2 cup strawberries
Meal 3 6:00pm	7-8oz lean ground beef with teriyaki sauce 2 cups vegetables with ranch dressing
Snack 2 8:30 or 9:00pm	4-5oz chicken with jerk sauce 1 cup vegetables with balsamic dressing

EATING PLAN 2

This is an example a fat loss diet for a female who is moderately active and can follow a low-carb diet.

The portion sizes are smaller as females usually do not eat as much. She would eat 3 meals a day with 2 snacks and have a cheat meal with carbs every 4th or 5th day.

If you have a hard time giving up carbs then add 1/2 cup to your lunch. If you don't eat much for breakfast, you can have Snack 1 at 8:00 a.m., then have Meal 1 as snack 2 at 3:00 p.m. Please see next page.

Meal 1 8:00am	1 whole egg with 1 slice cheese 1 serving medium apple
Meal 2 12:00pm	3-4oz chicken breast with sauce of your choice 1 to 1.5 cups of vegetables with dressing of your choice
Snack 1 3:00pm	1/2 cup protein powder 1 cup natural yogurt 1/2 cup blueberries
Meal 3 6:00pm	3-4oz salmon with teriyaki sauce 1 to 1.5 cups of vegetables with dressing of your choice
Snack 2 8:30 or 9:00pm	2-3oz tofu serving with soya sauce 1 cup vegetables with salad dressing of your choice or 1/4 cup of unsalted nuts of your choice

5 HEALTHY MEALS UNDER 400 CALORIES

Keeping fit is all about keeping the calories in check. Here are 5 healthy meals under 400 calories.

Eat well and enjoy!

MEAL 1

LOW FAT TURKEY SLOPPY JOES

Cook time: 30 minutes

Sandwiches: 4

Servings: 6

INGREDIENTS

1 lb lean ground turkey

$2/3$ cup onion

$1/2$ cup green pepper

2 jalapeno peppers

1 cup no-salt-added ketchup

2 tablespoons brown sugar

2 tablespoons Worcestershire sauce

1 tablespoon garlic powder

2 tablespoons chili powder

1 tablespoon mustard powder

$1/4$ teaspoon salt substitute

2 tablespoons extra virgin olive oil

DIRECTIONS

1. Remove seeds from jalapeno peppers and dice.

2. Dice onion and green pepper.

3. Sauté onion, jalapenos and green pepper then set aside.

4. Cook ground turkey crumbling into little pieces.

5. Drain and return to pan.

6. Over med-high heat add all of the ingredients into the pan.

7. Stir mixture for 3-5 minute.

8. Lower heat to low and simmer for 5-10 min to fuse flavors.

9. Serve on either crusty rolls or hamburger buns.

10. Leave out the jalapeno if you don't like it hot. If you do throw in a few more.

11. Additions: Try adding diced tomatoes or olives and top with cheese if you so desire.

Per serving: Calories 241.5 | Fat 11.2 g | Cholesterol 52.2 mg | Sodium 154.8 mg | Carbohydrate 21 g | Protein 16.8 g

MEAL 2

OVEN-FRIED CHICKEN CHIMICHANGAS

Cook time: 45 minutes

Servings: 6

INGREDIENTS

$\frac{2}{3}$ cup picante sauce or $\frac{2}{3}$ cup your favorite salsa

1 teaspoon ground cumin

$\frac{1}{2}$ teaspoon dried oregano leaves, crushed

1 $\frac{1}{2}$ cups cooked chicken, chopped

1 cup shredded cheddar cheese

2 green onions, chopped with some tops (about 1/4 cup)

6 (8 inch) flour tortillas

2 tablespoons margarine, melted

shredded cheddar cheese, for serving

chopped green onion, for serving

picante sauce, for serving

DIRECTIONS

1. Mix chicken, picante sauce or salsa, cumin, oregano, cheese and onions.

2. Place about 1/4 cup of the chicken mixture in the center of each tortilla.

3. Fold opposite sides over filling.

4. Roll up from bottom and place seam-side down on a baking sheet.

5. Brush with melted margarine.

6. Bake at 400°F for 25 minutes or until golden.

7. Garnish with additional cheese and green onion and serve salsa on the side.

Per serving: Calories 353.9 | Fat 16.8 g | Cholesterol 46 mg | Sodium 717.9 mg | Carbohydrate 31.5 g | Protein 18.7 g

MEAL 3

LEMON GRILLED SALMON WITH CORN SALAD

Cook time: 22 minutes

Yields: 4 servings

INGREDIENTS

1 $\frac{1}{2}$ cups corn kernels, cooked and cooled

$\frac{1}{3}$ cup sweet red pepper, chopped

$\frac{1}{4}$ cup chives, snipped

3 tablespoons fresh basil, thinly sliced

2 tablespoons pure maple syrup

2 tablespoons lemon juice

$\frac{1}{4}$ teaspoon salt

2 teaspoons lemon peel, finely shredded

1 teaspoon ground cumin

$\frac{1}{2}$ teaspoon salt

$\frac{1}{4}$ teaspoon black pepper

16 -20 ounces salmon fillets, 4 fillets each fillet weighing between 4 to 5 ounces, fresh skinless

1 $1\frac{1}{2}$ cups fresh blueberries

nonstick cooking spray

lemon slice (optional)

DIRECTIONS

1. For the corn salad: In bowl combine corn, sweet pepper, chives, basil, maple syrup, lemon juice, and the 1/4 teaspoon of salt.

2. For the salmon seasoning mixture: In small bowl, combine lemon peel, cumin, the 1/2 teaspoon salt, and the black pepper.

3. Lightly coat both sides of salmon with nonstick spray.

4. Sprinkle seasoning mixture over salmon fillets.

5. For charcoal grill, grill salmon fillets on the rack of an uncovered grill directly over medium coals for 8 to 12 minutes or until fish flakes easily when tested with a fork, carefully turning once halfway through grilling.

6. For gas grill, preheat grill. Reduce heat to medium. Place salmon fillets on grill rack over heat. Cover and grill as above.

6.Sprinkle a bit of paprika on the salmon.

7. Mix blueberries into the corn salad and serve grilled salmon with corn salad.

8. Garnish with lemon slices and/or fresh basil sprigs.

Per serving: Calories 318.7 | Fat 6.3 g | Cholesterol 51.6 mg | Sodium 527.4 mg | Carbohydrate 42.4 g | Protein 27.6 g

MEAL 4

Parmesan-Crusted Chicken With Arugula Salad

Cook time: 30 minutes

Servings: 4

INGREDIENTS

1 tablespoon Dijon mustard, divided

1 tablespoon extra virgin olive oil, divided

$\frac{1}{2}$ teaspoon chopped fresh thyme

4 (6 ounce) boneless skinless chicken breast halves

salt & freshly ground black pepper, to taste

$\frac{1}{2}$ cup freshly grated parmesan cheese, divided (you can use store-bought in a pinch)

$\frac{1}{2}$ teaspoon water

4 cups packed arugula (you can use a spring mix)

1 cup cherry tomatoes, halved

DIRECTIONS

1. Preheat the oven to 475 degrees.

2. In a small bowl, whisk 2 teaspoons of the mustard with 2 teaspoons of the olive oil and the thyme.

3. Season the chicken breasts, on both sides, with salt and pepper - then brush them all over with the mustard mixture.

4. Pat about 2 T. of the parmesan on each chicken breast (both sides) - it should take about 1/2 cup total for all 4 breasts.

5. Transfer the chicken breasts to a rimmed baking sheet.

6. Bake the chicken on the top shelf of the oven for about 15 minutes, or until just cooked through and nicely browned.

7. Meanwhile, in a salad bowl, combine the remaining 1 teaspoon each of mustard and oil; then stir in the water.

8. Add the arugula (or spring mix lettuce) and tomatoes. Season with salt and pepper and toss well.

9. Spoon the salad onto plates, top with the chicken and enjoy!

Per serving: Calories 291.9 | Fat 11.7 g | Cholesterol 119.9 mg | Sodium 438.4 mg | Carbohydrate 2.9 g | Protein 41.9 g

Meal 5

ZUCCHINI BEEF SKILLET

Cook time: 30 minutes

Serves: 4

INGREDIENTS

1 lb ground beef

1 chopped onion

$\frac{1}{2}$ chopped pepper

1 $\frac{1}{2}$ teaspoons salt

$\frac{1}{4}$ teaspoon pepper

1 teaspoon chili powder

3 cups sliced zucchini

1 (14 ounce) can diced tomatoes

$\frac{1}{2}$ cup water

DIRECTIONS

1. Saute onion and pepper.

2. Add ground beef and cook until brown.

3. Add remaining ingredients, cover, and simmer 15 minutes or until veggies are tender.

Per serving: Calories 290.8 | Fat 17.6 g | Cholesterol 77.1 mg | Sodium 972.4 mg | Carbohydrate 9.8 g | Protein 23.5 g

TRAINING GUIDELINES

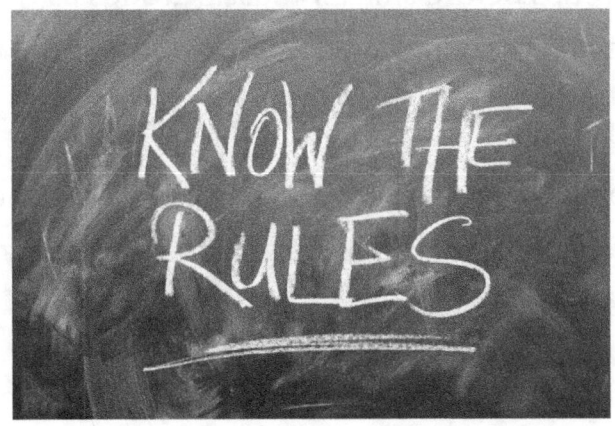

Read and memorize this before you start your training program.

1. Always practice good form. A good controlled set will recruit more muscle fibers verses throwing the weights around.

2. Do one warm up set with a lighter weight. This will allow you to practice the exercise and execute good form for the next sets.

3. Lower the weight in a controlled manner. The lowering part of the rep is called the negative (eccentric) portion. More control in the lowering portion will recruit more muscle fibers.

4. Breathe out with force. Never hold your breath during a set. Your muscles need oxygen to keep working and to expel carbon dioxide. A red face does not look attractive.

5. Know when to stop. Sometimes it is not good to push beyond failure. Pushing yourself to hard all the time can lead to injuries.

6. Record your weights in a book to track your progress. This is how to track your progress.

7. Do large muscle groups before smaller muscle groups as they require the most energy. Doing biceps before training your back is detrimental to your back workout as your arms will fatigue first.

8. Always set goals before you start any training program. Whether it be to lose 5lb, 10lbs, or to bench press your body weight. This will give you more purpose and will help you reach your goal.

9. Try not to grunt or scream when you do your set or reps. You're not auditioning for Tarzan.

10. If you are unsure of any exercises just look them up in the internet.

11. Weigh yourself once a week at the same time and day. Preferably in the morning before you eat breakfast.

WHAT ARE YOUR GOALS

What are your goals?

Do you want to lose 5lbs, 10lbs, or run a 5K?

Write down some of your goals below. List 2 short and long term goals.

Remember to be realistic as Rome was not built in a day.

1.

2.

3.

TWO WEEK FAT LOSS TRAINING PROGRAM – BEGINNER

Are you a coach potato or have are just starting an exercise regiment?

If you answered yes, just follow this two week program as a warm up. Then proceed to the eight week training program after.

Week 1

Sunday: Rest or walking for 20 minutes

Monday: Workout 1 (full body workout)

Tuesday: Rest

Wednesday: Cardio + core (abs)

Thursday: Workout 2 (full body workout)

Friday: Rest

Saturday: Cardio + core (abs)

Monday

Workout 1

1. Warm up for 5-6 minutes on a cardio machine

2. Lat pull down to front – 1x12, 1x10, 1x8 reps

3. Machine leg press – 1x12, 1x10, 1x8 reps

4. Machine back row – 1x12, 1x10, 1x8 reps

5. Machine bench press – 1x12, 1x10, 1x8 reps

6. Lying prone machine hamstring curls – 1x12, 1x10, 1x8 reps

7. Machine shoulder press – 1x12, 1x10, 1x8 reps

8. Seated adductor machine – 1x15, 1x12, 1x10 reps

9. Cool down for 5-6 minutes on a cardio machine

10. Static stretching or use my stretching app

https://goo.gl/RLSCHo

Wednesday

Cardio – 25 minutes

1. Bike – 12.5 minutes

2. Treadmill – 12.5 minutes

Core

1. Bird dogs - 1 x12, 1x12 reps

2. Seated leg lifts – 1x15, 1x15 for each side

3. Cable crunches - 1x15, 1x15 reps

4. Standing medicine ball twists – 1 minute

Thursday

Workout 2

1. Warm up for 5-6 minutes on a cardio machine

2. Reverse grip bar pull downs – 1x15, 1x12, 1x10 reps

3. Seated machine leg extensions – 1x15, 1x12, 1x10 reps

4. Pulley low grip back rows – 1x15, 1x12, 1x10 reps

5. Flat dumbbell chest fly – 1x15, 1x12, 1x10 reps

6. Seated upright hamstring curls – 1x15, 1x12, 1x10 reps

7. Dumbbell side laterals – 1x15, 1x12, 1x10 reps

8. Seal jacks – 1x15, 1x15 reps

9. Machine triceps extension – 1x15, 1x12, 1x10 reps

10. Machine biceps curls – 1x15, 1x10 reps

11. Cool down for 5-6 minutes on a cardio machine

12. Static stretching or use my stretching app

https://goo.gl/RLSCHo

Saturday

Cardio – 25 minutes

1. Elliptical – 12.5 minutes

2. Rowing – 12.5 minutes

Core

1. Hold superman – 1x15, 1x15 seconds

2. Standing bicycle crunches – 1x15, 1x15 reps

3. Oblique cable twists – 1x15, 1x15 each side

Week 2

Sunday: Rest or walking for 20 minutes

Monday: Workout 1 (same as week 1)

Tuesday: Rest

Wednesday: Cardio + core (same workout as week 1)

Thursday: Workout 2 (same as week 1)

Friday: Rest

Saturday: Cardio + core (same workout as week 1)

EIGHT WEEK FAT LOSS PROGRAM FOR MEN

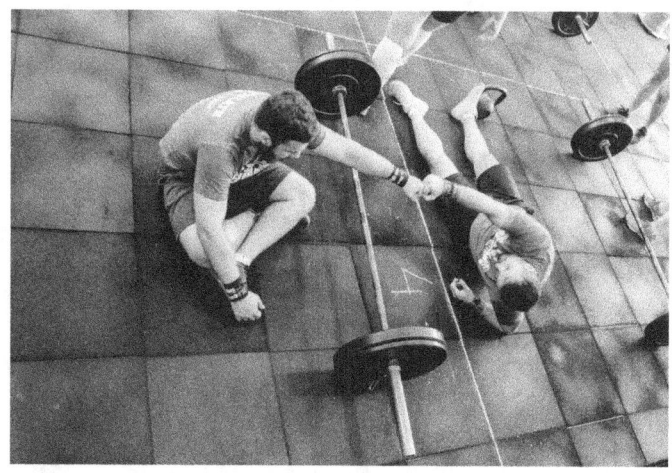

If you have completed the two week warm up program, you are now ready to start the eight week training program.

If you are not a beginner, then jump right into this program. The program is just a base for you to follow. Level 1(still a beginner) can follow the program. Level 2(advanced) can add an extra set to each exercise.

Bring a towel and get ready to sweat!

Week 1: Heavy Week

1. Figure out your 1RM (rep max) and then go up to 90% of your 1 RM for your last set.

- a 200lb bench press would be 180lbs for 4 on your last set

2. Figure out your basal metabolic rate (BMR) and make sure it matches your caloric intake.

3. There will be no caloric deficit because as each week progresses; there will be an increase in energy out put.

4. Always do a 5-8 minute warm up and 5-8 minute cooldown before and after every training session. This should include static stretching after your workout sessions.

5. If you are unsure of any exercise, just look it up on the internet.

6. Rest 40-60 seconds in between all sets and exercises.

7. Go to failure on the last set and record all your weights.

8. Use ascending pyramiding for all set and exercises throughout this program.

Sunday: Rest

Monday: Back+ shoulders+ traps + cardio

Tuesday: Cardio+core

Wednesday: Quadriceps+hamstrings+calves

Thursday: Rest

Friday: Chest+biceps+triceps+forearms+cardio

Saturday: Cardio+core

Monday

Back

1. Pulldown to front - 1x10, 1x8, 1x6 reps

2. Barbell back rows - 1x10, 1x8, 1x6 reps

3. Reverse grip pulldowns - 1x10, 1x8, 1x6 reps

4. Machine back rows - 1x10, 1x18, 1x6 reps

Shoulders

1. Machine shoulder press - 1x10, 1x8, 1x6 reps

2. Bent over rear dumbbell laterals - 1x10, 1x8, 1x6 reps

3. Bar upright rows - 1x10, 1x8, 1x6 reps

Traps

1. Barbell front shrugs - 1x10, 1x8 reps

2. Behind the body barbell shrugs - 1x10, 1x8 reps

Cardio

1. Bike or treadmill - 20 minutes

Tuesday

Cardio - 25 minutes

1. Bike - 5 minutes

2. Treadmill - 10 minutes

3. Rowing machine - 10 minutes (HIIT intervals)

Core

1. Land swimming - 1x15, 1x15 seconds

2. Bench V-up - 1x15, 1x15, 1x15 reps

3. Dumbbell Side tilts - 1x15, 1x15 each side

4. Elbow plank - 1 x 30 seconds

Wednesday

Quadriceps

1. Plate loader leg press - 1x10, 1x8, 1x6, 1x4 reps

2. Leg extensions - 1x10,, 1x8, 1x6, 1x4 reps

3. Back squats - 1x10, 1x8, 1x6, 1x4 reps

Hamstrings

1. Lying leg curls - 1x10, 1x8, 1x6 reps

2. Stiff legged deadlifts (bar) - 1x10, 1x8, 1x6 reps

Calves

1. Seated calf raises - 1x12, 1 x10, 1x8 reps

2. Standing machine calf raises - 1x12, 1x10, 1x8 reps

Friday

Chest

1. Decline bar bench press- 1x10, 1x8, 1x6 reps

2. Incline dumbbell bench press - 1x10, 1x8, 1x6 reps

3. Incline dumbbell fly - 1x10, 1x8, 1x6 reps

Biceps

1. Seated alternate dumbbell curls - 1x10, 1x8, 1x6 reps

2. Machine preacher curls - 1x10, 1x8, 1x6 reps

Triceps

1. Rope pulley pushdowns - 1x10, 1x8, 1x6 reps

2. One arm overhead dumbbell extensions - 1x10, 1x8 reps

3. Lying dumbbell triceps extensions - 1x10, 1x8 reps

Forearms

1. Incline partial hammer curls - 1x10, 1x8 reps

2. Behind- the- back wrist curls - 1x10, 1x8 reps

Cardio

1. Bike - 20 minutes

Saturday

Cardio

-same cardio as Tuesday

Core

-same core as Tuesday

Week 2: Light Medium Week

1. Go up to 70% or your 1RM (rep max).

- A 200 lb bench press would be 140 for 10 reps on the last set

2. Do not go to failure on any set.

3. Rest 30-40 seconds between all sets and reps.

Sunday: Rest or light walking

Monday: Chest+quads+adductors+abductors

Tuesday: Cardio+core

Wednesday: Back+hamstrings+biceps+forearms+cardio

Thursday: Rest

Friday: Shoulders+traps+triceps+claves+cardio

Saturday: Cardio+core

Monday

Chest

1. Incline bar chest press – 1x15, 1x12, 1x10 reps

2. Cable crossovers- 1x15, 1x12, 1x10 reps

3. Dumbbell pullovers- 1x15, 1x12, 1x10 reps

Quadriceps

1. Leg extensions- 1x15, 1x12, 1x10, 1x10 reps

2. Plie dumbbell squats- 1x15, 1x12, 1x10, 1x10 reps

3. Seated adductor machine – 1x15, 1x12, 1x10 reps

4. Seated abductor machine- 1x15, 1x12, 1x10 reps

Tuesday

Cardio – 30 minutes

1. Bike- 10 minutes

2. Treadmill- 10 minutes

3. Rowing machine- 10 minutes(HIIT intervals)

Core

1. Good mornings- 1x12, 1x12 reps

2. Pulley wood chops- 1x12, 1x12 reps

3. Swiss ball leg lifts- 1x15, 1x15, 1x15 reps

4. Legs on Swiss ball crunches- 1x15, 1x15, 1x15 reps

Wednesday

Back

1. Bar deadlifts 1x15, 1x12, 1x10 reps

2. Close grip v-bar pulldowns- 1x15, 1x12, 1x10 reps

3. One arm dumbbell back rows – 1x15, 1x12, 1x10 reps

4. Rope pulley pullovers- 1x15, 1x12, 1x10 reps

Hamstrings

1.Standing leg curls- 1x15, 1x12, 1x10 reps

2. Lying leg curls – 1x15, 1x12, 1x10 reps

Biceps

1.Standing pulley biceps curls- 1x15, 1x12, 1x10 reps

2. Incline dumbbell curls – 1x15, 1x12, 1x10 reps

Forearms

1. Reverse grip pulldowns- 1x15, 1x10 reps

2. Cross the bench flexor curls-1x15, 1x10 reps

Cardio- 20 minutes

1.Bike or elliptical

Friday

Shoulders

1.Standing front barbell press-1x15,1x12,1x10 reps

2. Seated bent over laterals-1x15, 1x12, 1x10 reps

3. Standing side cable laterals – 1x15, 1x12, 1x10 reps

Traps

1.Dumbbell shrugs- 1x15, 1x12, 1x10 reps

Triceps

1.Close grip bench presses- 1x15, 1x12, 1x10 reps

2. One arm dumbbell overhead extensions – 1x15, 1x12 reps

3. Dip machine – 1x15, 1x12 reps

Calves

1.Standing machine calf raises- 1x15, 1x12, 1x10 reps

2. Seated calf raises- 1x15, 1x12, 1x10 reps

Cardio-20 minutes

1. Elliptical or bike

Saturday

Cardio- 25 minutes

-same cardio as Tuesday

Core

-same core as Tuesday

Week 3: Heavy Week

1. Same workout as week 1.

2. Increase all weights by 5-10lbs on all exercises from week 1.

3. Go to failure on all last set for all exercises.

4. Rest 40-60 seconds in between all sets and reps.

Sunday: Rest or 20 minute light walk

Monday: Back+shoulders+traps+cardio

Tuesday: Cardio+core

Wednesday: Quads+hamstrings+calves

Thursday: Rest

Friday: Chest+biceps+triceps+forearms+cardio

Saturday: Cardio+core

Monday

Back

1.Reverse grip pulldowns – 1x12, 1x10, 1x8 reps

2. Barbell back rows – 1x12, 1x10, 1x8 reps

3. Pulldown to front - 1x12, 1x10, 1x8 reps

4. Machine back rows - 1x12, 1x10, 1x8 reps

Shoulders

1.Machine shoulder press - 1x12, 1x10, 1x8 reps

2. Bar upright row - 1x12, 1x10, 1x8 reps

3. Bent over dumbbell laterals - 1x12, 1x10, 1x8 reps

Traps

1.Barbell front shrugs - 1x12, 1x10 reps

2. Barbell behind the body shrugs - 1x12, 1x10 reps

Cardio

1.Treadmile or bike – 20 minutes

Tuesday

Cardio - 30 minutes

1. Elliptical - 10 minutes

2. Bike - 10 minutes

3. Treadmill - 10 minutes (HIIT intervals)

Core

1. Single prone leg lifts - 1x12, 1x12 each leg

2. Elbow plank – 30 seconds x2

3. V-sit holds – 30 seconds x2

4. Side planks – 30 seconds x1 each side

Wednesday

Quadriceps

1. Back barbell squats - 1x12, 1x10, 1x8, 1x6 reps

2. Leg extensions - 1x12, 1x10, 1x8, 1x6 reps

3. Plate loader leg press - 1x12, 1x10, 1x8, 1x6 reps

Hamstrings

1. Stiff legged deadlifts - 1x12, 1x10, 1x8 reps

2. Lying leg curls - 1x12, 1x10, 1x8, 1x6 reps

Calves

1. Standing weighted calf raises- 1x15, 1x12, 1x10 reps

2. Seated calf raises - 1x15, 1x12, 1x10 reps

Friday

Chest

1. Incline dumbbell bench press - 1x12, 1x10, 1x8 reps

2. Decline barbell bench press - 1x12, 1x10, 1x8 reps

3. Incline dumbbell fly - 1x12, 1x10, 1x8 reps

Biceps

1. Machine preacher curl - 1x12, 1x10, 1x8 reps

2. Seated alternate dumbbell curls - 1x12, 1x10, 1x8 reps

Triceps

1. Lying dumbbell triceps extensions - 1x12, 1x10, 1x8 reps

2. One arm overhead triceps extensions - 1x12, 1x10 reps

3. Rope pulley pushdowns - 1x12, 1x10 reps

Forearms

1. Behind the body curls - 1x12, 1x10 reps

2. Incline partial hammer curls - 1x12, 1x10 reps

Cardio

1. Treadmill or bike - 20 minutes

Saturday

Cardio

-same cardio as Tuesday

Core

-same core as Tuesday

Week 4: Light medium week

1. Same workout as week 2 but higher rep scheme.

2. Do not go to failure on any set.

3. Use same weights as week 2.

4. 3. Rest 30-40 seconds between all sets and reps.

Sunday: Rest or light walking

Monday: Chest+quads+adductors+abductors

Tuesday: Cardio+core

Wednesday: Back+hamstrings+biceps+forearms+cardio

Thursday: Rest

Friday: Shoulders+traps+triceps+claves+cardio

Saturday: Cardio+core

Monday

Chest

1. Dumbbell pullovers- 1x20,1x15,1 x12 reps

2. Incline bar chest press – 1x20,1x15,1 x12 reps

3. Cable crossovers- 1x20,1x15,1 x12 reps

Quadriceps

1. Seated adductor machine – 1x20,1x15,1 x12 reps

2. Seated abductor machine- 1x20,1x15,1 x12 reps

3. Leg extensions- 1x20,1x15,1 x12, 1x10 reps

4. Plie dumbbell squats- 1x20,1x15,1 x12, 1x10 reps

Tuesday

Cardio - 35 minutes

1. Bike - 15 minutes

2. Elliptical - 10 minutes

3. Treadmill or run outside - 10 minutes (HIIT intervals)

Core

1. Bird dogs - 1x12, 1x12 each side

2. Stability ball passes - 1x10, 1x10, 1x10 reps

3. Standing Russian ball twists - 1 minute x 1

Wednesday

Back

1. Rope pulley pullovers- 1x20,1x15,1 x12 reps

2.Close grip v-bar pulldowns- 1x20,1x15,1 x12 reps

3. One arm dumbbell back rows – 1x20,1x15,1 x12 reps

4. Bar deadlifts - 1x20,1x15,1 x12 reps

Hamstrings

1.. Lying leg curls – 1x20,1x15,1 x12 reps

2.Standing leg curls- 1x20,1x15,1 x12 reps

Biceps

1. Incline dumbbell curls – 1x20,1x15,1 x12 reps

2.Standing pulley biceps curls- 1x20,1x15,1 x12 reps

Forearms

1. Cross the bench flexor curls- 1x20,1x15 reps

2. Reverse grip pulldowns- 1x20,1x15 reps

Cardio- 20 minutes

1.Bike or treadmill

Friday

Shoulders

1. Standing side cable laterals – 1x20,1x15,1 x12 reps

2.Standing front barbell press-1x20,1x15,1 x12 reps

3. Seated bent over laterals-1x20,1x15,1 x12 reps

Traps

1.Dumbbell shrugs- 1x20,1x15,1 x12 reps

Triceps

1. Dip machine – 1x20,1x15,1 x12 reps

1.Close grip bench presses- 1x20,1x15 reps

2. One arm dumbbell overhead extensions – 1x20,1x15 reps

Calves

1. Seated calf raises- 1x20,1x15,1 x12 reps

2.Standing machine calf raises- 1x20,1x15,1x12 reps

Cardio-20 minutes

1. Elliptical or bike

Saturday

Cardio

- same cardio as Tuesday

Core

-same core as Tuesday

Week 5 : Heavy week

1. Figure out your 1RM (rep max) and then go up to 90% of your 1 RM for your last set.

2. Go to failure on your last set for each exercise.

3. Rest 40-60 seconds between all sets and reps.

Sunday: Rest or 20 minute light walk

Monday: Chest+shoulders+triceps+cardio

Tuesday: Cardio+core

Wednesday: Back+hamstrings+calves

Thursday: Rest

Friday: Quads+biceps+forearms+traps+cardio

Saturday: Cardio+core

Monday

Chest

1. Flat bar bench press - 1x10, 1x8, 1x6 reps

2. Incline bar bench press - 1x10, 1x8, 1x6 reps

3. Decline dumbbell fly - 1x10, 1x8, 1x6 reps

Shoulders

1. Dumbbell shoulder press - 1x10, 1x8, 1x6 reps

2. Dumbbell side laterals - 1x10, 1x8, 1x6 reps

3. Pulley rear delt face pulls - 1x10, 1x8, 1x6 reps

Triceps

1. Bar pulley pushdowns - 1x10, 1x8, 1x6 reps

2. Rope pulley overhead extensions - 1x10, 1x8, 1x6 reps

3. Partial mini dips - 1x10, 1x8, 1x6 reps

Cardio-25 minutes

1. Elliptical or bike

Tuesday

Cardio- 35 minutes

1. Treadmill - 10 minutes

2. Bike - 15 minutes

3. Elliptical - 10 minutes (HIIT intervals)

Core

1. Good mornings – 1x15, 1x15 reps

2. Jackknife sit ups – 1x15, 1x15, 1x15 reps

3. Side plank to reach under – 1x10, 1x10 each side

Wednesday

Back

1. Close grip low pulley row - 1x10, 1x8, 1x6 reps

2. Barbell back rows - 1x10, 1x8, 1x6 reps

3. Reverse grip pulldowns - 1x10, 1x8, 1x6 reps

4. Machine assissted chin-ups - 1x10, 1x8, 1x6 reps

Hamstrings

1. Seated leg curls - 1x10, 1x8, 1x6 reps

2. Dumbbell stiff legged deadlifts - 1x10, 1x8, 1x6 reps

Calves

1. Plate loader calf pushes - 1x10, 1x18, 1x6 reps

2. Seated calf raises - 1x10, 1x8, 1x6 reps

Friday

Quadriceps

1. Plate loader leg press - 1x10, 1x8, 1x6 reps

2. Back squats - 1x10, 1x8, 1x6 reps

3. Leg extensions - 1x10, 1x8, 1x6 reps

4. Machine leg press - 1x10, 1x8, 1x6 reps

Traps

1. Dumbbell shrugs - 1x10, 1x8, 1x6, reps

Biceps

1. Barbell biceps curls - 1x10, 1x8, 1x6 reps

2. Incline dumbbell biceps curls - 1x10, 1x8, 1x6 reps

Forearms

1. Dumbbell hammer curls - 1x10, 1x8 reps

2. Behind the body wrist curls - 1x10, 1x8 reps

Saturday

Cardio

-same cardio as Tuesday

Core

-same core as Tuesday

Week 6: Light medium week

1. Increase weights by 5lbs - 10 lbs on all weights from week 4.

2. Do not go to failure on any set.

3. Rest 30-40 seconds between all sets and reps.

Sunday: Rest or 20 minute walk

Monday: Chest+back+cardio

Tuesday: Cardio+core

Wednesday: Quads+shoulders+traps+calves

Thursday: Rest

Friday: Triceps+biceps+forearms+cardio

Saturday: Cardio+core

Monday

Chest

1. Flat dumbbell bench press - 1x15, 1x12, 1x10 reps

2. Machine chest fly - 1x15, 1x12, 1x10 reps

3. Incline dumbbell chest press - 1x15, 1x12, 1x10 reps

Back

1. Lat pulldown to front - 1x15, 1x12, 1x10 reps

2. Machine under grip pulldowns - 1x15, 1x12, 1x10 reps

3. Machine back row - 1x15, 1x12, 1x10 reps

4. T-bar rows - 1x15, 1x12, 1x10 reps

Cardio - 25 minutes

1. Treadmill or bike

Tuesday

Cardio - 40 minutes

1. Rowing - 15 minutes

2. Treadmill - 15 minutes

3. Bike - 10 minutes (HIIT intervals)

Core

1. Reverse hyperextensions on stability ball - 1x15, 1x15 reps

2. Scissor kicks - 1x15, 1x15, 1x15 reps

3. Dumbbell crunches - 1x15, 1x15, 1x15 reps

4. Standing pulley twists - 1x12, 1x12 each side

Wednesday

Quadriceps

1. Bulgarian split squats - 1x15, 1x12, 1x10 for each leg

2. Leg extensions - 1x15, 1x12, 1x10, 1x10 reps

3. Standing side to side lunges - 1x12, 1x12, 1x12 for each side

Shoulders

1. Seated dumbbell side laterals - 1x15, 1x12, 1x10 reps

2. Standing front dumbbell laterals - 1x15, 1x12, 1x10 reps

3. Bent over rear cable laterals - 1x15, 1x12, 1x10 reps

Traps

1. Barbell shrugs - 1x15, 1x12, 1x10 reps

Calves

1. Seated calf raises - 1x15, 1x12, 1x10 reps

2. Machine leg press calf pushes - 1x15, 1x12, 1x10 reps

Friday

Triceps

1. W-bar skull crushers - 1x15, 1x12, 1x10 reps

2. Two arm dumbbell overhead triceps extensions - 1x15, 1x12 reps

3. One arm dumbbell kickbacks - 1x15, 1x12 for each arm

Biceps

1. Standing dumbbell biceps alternate curls - 1x15, 1x12, 1x10 reps

2. Standing high pulley cable curls - 1x15, 1x12, 1x10 reps

Forearms

1. Extension cross the bench barbell reverse wrist curls - 1x15, 1x12 reps

2. Cross the bench barbell flexor wrist curls - 1x15, 1x12 reps

Cardio - 25 minutes

1. Bike or treadmill

Saturday

Cardio

-same as Tuesday

Core

-same as Tuesday

Week 7: Heavy week

1. Go up 5-10lbs on all exercises from week 5.

2. Go to failure on your last set for each exercise.

3. Rest 40-60 seconds between all sets and reps.

Sunday: Rest or 20 minute light walk

Monday: Chest+shoulders+triceps+cardio

Tuesday: Cardio+core

Wednesday: Back+hamstrings+calves

Thursday: Rest

Friday: Quads+biceps+forearms+traps+cardio

Saturday: Cardio+core

Monday

Chest

1. Incline bench press - 1x12, 1x10, 1x8 reps

2. Flat bench press - 1x12, 1x10, 1x8 reps

3. Decline dumbbell fly - 1x12, 1x10, 1x8 reps

Shoulders

1. Dumbbell side laterals - 1x12, 1x10, 1x8 reps

2. Dumbbell shoulder press - 1x12, 1x10, 1x8 reps

3. Pulley rear delt face pulls - 1x12, 1x10, 1x8 reps

Triceps

1. Partial mini dips - 1x12, 1x10, 1x8 reps

2. Rope pulley overhead triceps extensions - 1x12, 1x10 reps

3. Bar pulley pushdowns - 1x12, 1x10 reps

Cardio - 25 minutes

1. Treadmill or bike

Tuesday

Cardio - 40 minutes

1. Elliptical - 10 minutes

2. Bike - 20 minutes

3. Treadmill - 10 minutes (HIIT)

Core

1. Superman holds - 1x20, 1x20 seconds

2. Reverse crunches - 1x15, 1x15, 1x15 reps

3. Incline sit-ups - 1x15, 1x15, 1x15 reps

4. Standing holding dumbbell side tilts - 1x12, 1x12 each side

Wednesday

Back

1. Machine assisted chin-ups - 1x12, 1x10, 1x8 reps

2. Reverse grip pulldowns - 1x12, 1x10, 1x8 reps

3. Barbell back rows - 1x12, 1x10, 1x8 reps

4. Close grip pulley rows - 1x12, 1x10, 1x8 reps

Hamstrings

1. Dumbbell stiff legged deadlifts - 1x12, 1x10, 1x8 reps

2. Seated leg curls - 1x12, 1x10, 1x8 reps

Calves

1. Seated calf raises - 1x12, 1x10, 1x8 reps

2. Plate loader calf pushes - 1x12, 1x10, 1x8 reps

Friday

Quadriceps

1. Back squats - 1x12, 1x10, 1x8 reps

2. Plate loader leg press - 1x12, 1x10, 1x8 reps

3. Machine leg press - 1x12, 1x10, 1x8 reps

4. Leg extensions - 1x12, 1x10, 1x8 reps

Traps

1. Dumbbell shrugs - 1x12, 1x10, 1x8, 1x6 reps

Biceps

1. Incline dumbbell curls - 1x12, 1x10, 1x8 reps

2. Barbell biceps curls - 1x12, 1x10, 1x8 reps

Forearms

1. Behind the body back curls - 1x12, 1x10 reps

2. Dumbbell hammer curls - 1x12, 1x10 reps

Cardio - 25 minutes

1. Elliptical or treadmill

Saturday

Cardio- 40 minutes

- same as Tuesday

Core

-same as Tuesday

Week 8: Light Medium Week

1. Keep the weights the same from week 6.

2. Do not go to failure on any set.

3. Rest 30-40 seconds between all sets and reps.

Sunday: Rest or 20 minute walk

Monday: Chest+back+cardio

Tuesday: Cardio+core

Wednesday: Quads+shoulders+traps+calves

Thursday: Rest

Friday: Triceps+biceps+forearms+cardio

Saturday: Cardio+core

Monday

Chest

1. Incline dumbbell chest press - 1x20, 1x15, 1x10 reps

2. Machine chest fly - 1x20, 1x15, 1x10 reps

3. Flat dumbbell bench press - 1x20, 1x15, 1x10 reps

Back

1. Machine under grip pulldowns - 1x20, 1x15, 1x10 reps

2. T-bar back rows - 1x20, 1x15, 1x10 reps

3. Lat pulldown to front - 1x20, 1x15, 1x10 reps

4. Machine back row - 1x20, 1x15, 1x10 reps

Cardio - 25 minutes

1. Bike or run outside

Tuesday

Cardio-40 minutes

1. Treadmill - 20 minutes

2. Elliptical - 10 minutes

3. Rowing machine - 10 minutes (HIIT intervals)

Core

1. Single prone leg lifts - 1x15, 1x15 each side

2. Standing oblique twists with bar – 30 second x2

3. Bicycles crunches - 1x20, 1x20, 1x20 reps

Wednesday

Quadriceps

1. Leg extensions - 1x20, 1x15, 1x12, 1x10 reps

2. Bulgarian spilt squats - 1x15, 1x12, 1x10 each side

3. Standing side to side lunges - 1x15, 1x15, 1x15 each side

Shoulders

1. Front dumbbell laterals - 1x20, 1x15, 1x10 reps

2. Side dumbbell laterals - 1x20, 1x15, 1x10 reps

3. Bent over rear laterals - 1x20, 1x15, 1x10 reps

Traps

1. Barbell shrugs - 1x20, 1x15, 1x10 reps

Calves

1. Machine leg calf pushes - 1x20, 1x15, 1x10 reps

2. Seated calf raises - 1x20, 1x15, 1x10 reps

Friday

Triceps

1. W-bar skull crushers - 1x20, 1x15, 1x10 reps

2. One arm dumbbell triceps kickbacks - 1x20, 1x15 reps

3. Two arm dumbbell overhead triceps extensions - 1x20, 1x15 reps

Biceps

1. Standing dumbbell alternate curls - 1x20, 1x15, 1x10 reps

2. Standing high pulley cable curls - 1x20, 1x15, 1x10 reps

Forearms

1. Cross the bench barbell flexor curls - 1x20, 1x15 reps

2. Extension cross the bench barbell reverse wrist curls - 1x20, 1x15 reps

Cardio-25 minutes

1. Treadmill

Saturday

Cardio

-same as Tuesday

Core

-same as Tuesday

EIGHT WEEK FAT LOSS TRAINING PROGRAM FOR WOMEN

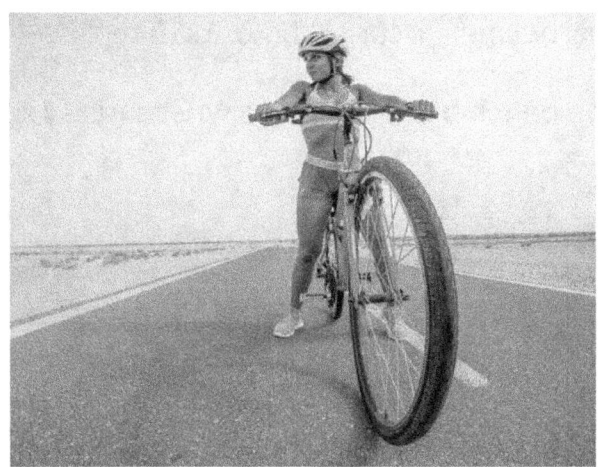

If you have completed the two week warm up program, you are now ready for the eight week training program.

If you are not a beginner, then jump right into this program.

Remember, if the volume of sets and repetitions are too much, then just reduce the amount to suit your individual needs.

Bring a towel and get ready to sweat!

Week 1: Heavy Week

1. Figure out your 1RM (rep max) and then go up to 90% of your 1 RM for your last set.

- a 200lb bench press would be 180lbs for 4 on your last set

2. Figure out your basal metabolic rate (BMR) and make sure it matches your caloric intake.

- if you are eating under your BMR and feel full do not eat extra calories

3. There will be no caloric deficit because as each week progresses; there will be an increase in energy out put.

4. Always do a 5-8 minute warm up and 5-8 minute cooldown before and after every training session. This should include static stretching after your workout sessions.

5. If you are unsure of any exercise, just look it up on the internet.

6. Rest 40-60 seconds in between all sets and exercises.

7. Go to failure on the last set and record all your weights.

8. Use ascending pyramiding for all set and exercises throughout this program.

Sunday: Rest

Monday: Back+ shoulders+ cardio

Tuesday: Cardio+core

Wednesday: Quadriceps+hamstrings+calves

Thursday: Rest

Friday: Chest+biceps+triceps+cardio

Saturday: Cardio+core

Monday

Back

1. Pulldown to front - 1x10, 1x8, 1x6 reps

2. Barbell back rows - 1x10, 1x8, 1x6 reps

3. Reverse grip pulldowns - 1x10, 1x8, 1x6 reps

4. Machine back rows - 1x10, 1x18, 1x6 reps

Shoulders

1. Machine shoulder press - 1x10, 1x8, 1x6 reps

2. Bent over rear dumbbell laterals - 1x10, 1x8, 1x6 reps

3. Bar upright rows - 1x10, 1x8, 1x6 reps

Cardio

1. Bike or treadmill - 20 minutes

Tuesday

Cardio - 25 minutes

1. Bike - 5 minutes

2. Treadmill - 10 minutes

3. Rowing machine - 10 minutes (HIIT intervals)

Core

1. Land swimming - 1x15, 1x15 seconds

2. Bench V-up - 1x15, 1x15, 1x15 reps

3. Dumbbell Side tilts - 1x15, 1x15 each side

4. Elbow plank - 1 x 30 seconds

Wednesday

Quadriceps

1. Plate loader leg press - 1x10, 1x8, 1x6, 1x4 reps

2. Leg extensions - 1x10,, 1x8, 1x6, 1x4 reps

3. Back squats - 1x10, 1x8, 1x6, 1x4 reps

Hamstrings

1. Lying leg curls - 1x10, 1x8, 1x6 reps

2. Stiff legged deadlifts (bar) - 1x10, 1x8, 1x6 reps

Calves

1. Seated calf raises - 1x12, 1 x10, 1x8 reps

2. Standing machine calf raises - 1x12, 1x10, 1x8 reps

Friday

Chest

1. Decline bar bench press- 1x10, 1x8, 1x6 reps

2. Incline dumbbell bench press - 1x10, 1x8, 1x6 reps

3. Incline dumbbell fly - 1x10, 1x8, 1x6 reps

Biceps

1. Seated alternate dumbbell curls - 1x10, 1x8, 1x6 reps

2. Machine preacher curls - 1x10, 1x8, 1x6 reps

Triceps

1. Rope pulley pushdowns - 1x10, 1x8, 1x6 reps

2. One arm overhead dumbbell extensions - 1x10, 1x8 reps

3. Lying dumbbell triceps extensions - 1x10, 1x8 reps

Cardio

1. Bike - 20 minutes

Saturday

Cardio

-same cardio as Tuesday

Core

-same core as Tuesday

Week 2: Light Medium Week

1. Go up to 70% or your 1RM (rep max).

- A 200 lb bench press would be 140 for 10 reps on the last set

2. Do not go to failure on any set.

3. Rest 30-40 seconds between all sets and reps.

Sunday: Rest

Monday: Chest+quads+adductors+abductors

Tuesday: Cardio+core

Wednesday: Back+hamstrings+biceps+cardio

Thursday: Rest

Friday: Shoulders+triceps+glutes+claves+cardio

Saturday: Cardio+core

Monday

Chest

1. Incline bar chest press – 1x15, 1x12, 1x10 reps

2. Cable crossovers- 1x15, 1x12, 1x10 reps

3. Dumbbell pullovers- 1x15, 1x12, 1x10 reps

Quadriceps

1. Leg extensions- 1x15, 1x12, 1x10, 1x10 reps

2. Plie dumbbell squats- 1x15, 1x12, 1x10, 1x10 reps

3. Seated adductor machine – 1x15, 1x12, 1x10 reps

4. Seated abductor machine- 1x15, 1x12, 1x10 reps

Tuesday

Cardio – 25 minutes

1. Bike- 10 minutes

2. Treadmill- 10 minutes

3. Rowing machine- 10 minutes(HIIT intervals)

Core

1. Good mornings- 1x12, 1x12 reps

2. Pulley wood chops- 1x12, 1x12 reps

3. Swiss ball leg lifts- 1x15, 1x15, 1x15 reps

4. Legs on Swiss ball crunches- 1x15, 1x15, 1x15 reps

Wednesday

Back

1. Bar deadlifts 1x15, 1x12, 1x10 reps

2. Close grip v-bar pulldowns- 1x15, 1x12, 1x10 reps

3. One arm dumbbell back rows – 1x15, 1x12, 1x10 reps

4. Rope pulley pullovers- 1x15, 1x12, 1x10 reps

Hamstrings

1.Standing leg curls- 1x15, 1x12, 1x10 reps

2. Lying leg curls – 1x15, 1x12, 1x10 reps

Biceps

1.Standing pulley biceps curls- 1x15, 1x12, 1x10 reps

2. Incline dumbbell curls – 1x15, 1x12, 1x10 reps

Cardio- 20 minutes

1.Bike or elliptical

Friday

Shoulders

1.Standing front barbell press-1x15,1x12,1x10 reps

2. Seated bent over laterals-1x15, 1x12, 1x10 reps

3. Standing side cable laterals – 1x15, 1x12, 1x10 reps

Triceps

1.Close grip bench presses- 1x15, 1x12, 1x10 reps

2. One arm dumbbell overhead extensions – 1x15, 1x12 reps

3. Dip machine – 1x15, 1x12 reps

Glutes

1. Table top glute kickbacks – 1x15, 1x15, 1x15 each leg

Calves

1.Standing machine calf raises- 1x15, 1x12, 1x10 reps

2. Seated calf raises- 1x15, 1x12, 1x10 reps

Cardio-20 minutes

1. Elliptical or bike

Saturday

Cardio

-same cardio as Tuesday

Core

-same core as Tuesday

Week 3: Heavy Week

1. Same workout as week 1.

2. Increase all weights by 2.5-5lbs on all exercises from week 1.

3. Go to failure on all last set for all exercises.

4. Rest 40-60 seconds in between all sets and reps.

Sunday: Rest

Monday: Back+shoulders+cardio

Tuesday: Cardio+core

Wednesday: Quads+hamstrings+calves

Thursday: Rest

Friday: Chest+biceps+triceps+cardio

Saturday: Cardio+core

Monday

Back

1.Reverse grip pulldowns – 1x12, 1x10, 1x8 reps

2. Barbell back rows – 1x12, 1x10, 1x8 reps

3. Pulldown to front - 1x12, 1x10, 1x8 reps

4. Machine back rows - 1x12, 1x10, 1x8 reps

Shoulders

1.Machine shoulder press - 1x12, 1x10, 1x8 reps

2. Bar upright row - 1x12, 1x10, 1x8 reps

3. Bent over dumbbell laterals - 1x12, 1x10, 1x8 reps

Cardio

1.Treadmile or bike – 20 minutes

Tuesday

Cardio - 30 minutes

1. Elliptical - 10 minutes

2. Bike - 10 minutes

3. Treadmill - 10 minutes (HIIT intervals)

Core

1. Single prone leg lifts - 1x12, 1x12 each leg

2. Elbow plank – 30 seconds x2

3. V-sit holds – 30 seconds x2

4. Side planks – 30 seconds x1 each side

Wednesday

Quadriceps

1. Back barbell squats - 1x12, 1x10, 1x8, 1x6 reps

2. Leg extensions - 1x12, 1x10, 1x8, 1x6 reps

3. Plate loader leg press - 1x12, 1x10, 1x8, 1x6 reps

Hamstrings

1. Stiff legged deadlifts - 1x12, 1x10, 1x8 reps

2. Lying leg curls - 1x12, 1x10, 1x8, 1x6 reps

Calves

1. Standing weighted calf raises- 1x15, 1x12, 1x10 reps

2. Seated calf raises - 1x15, 1x12, 1x10 reps

Friday

Chest

1. Incline dumbbell bench press - 1x12, 1x10, 1x8 reps

2. Decline barbell bench press - 1x12, 1x10, 1x8 reps

3. Incline dumbbell fly - 1x12, 1x10, 1x8 reps

Biceps

1. Machine preacher curl - 1x12, 1x10, 1x8 reps

2. Seated alternate dumbbell curls - 1x12, 1x10, 1x8 reps

Triceps

1. Lying dumbbell triceps extensions - 1x12, 1x10, 1x8 reps

2. One arm overhead triceps extensions - 1x12, 1x10 reps

3. Rope pulley pushdowns - 1x12, 1x10 reps

Forearms

1. Behind the body curls - 1x12, 1x10 reps

2. Incline partial hammer curls - 1x12, 1x10 reps

Cardio

1. Treadmile or bike - 20 minutes

Saturday

Cardio

-same cardio as Tuesday

Core

-same core as Tuesday

Week 4: Light medium week

1. Same workout as week 2 but higher rep scheme.

2. Do not go to failure on any set.

3. Use same weights as week 2.

4. 3. Rest 30-40 seconds between all sets and reps.

Sunday: Rest or light walking

Monday: Chest+quads+adductors+abductors

Tuesday: Cardio+core

Wednesday: Back+hamstrings+biceps+cardio

Thursday: Rest

Friday: Shoulders+triceps+glutes+claves+cardio

Saturday: Cardio+core

Monday

Chest

1. Dumbbell pullovers- 1x20,1x15,1 x12 reps

2. Incline bar chest press – 1x20,1x15,1 x12 reps

3. Cable crossovers- 1x20,1x15,1 x12 reps

Quadriceps

1. Seated adductor machine – 1x20,1x15,1 x12 reps

2. Seated abductor machine- 1x20,1x15,1 x12 reps

3. Leg extensions- 1x20,1x15,1 x12, 1x10 reps

4. Plie dumbbell squats- 1x20,1x15,1 x12, 1x10 reps

Tuesday

Cardio - 30 minutes

1. Bike - 15 minutes

2. Elliptical - 10 minutes

3. Treadmill or run outside - 10 minutes (HIIT intervals)

Core

1. Bird dogs - 1x12, 1x12 each side

2. Stability ball passes - 1x10, 1x10, 1x10 reps

3. Standing Russian ball twists - 1 minute x 1

Wednesday

Back

1. Rope pulley pullovers- 1x20,1x15,1 x12 reps

2.Close grip v-bar pulldowns- 1x20,1x15,1 x12 reps

3. One arm dumbbell back rows – 1x20,1x15,1 x12 reps

4. Bar deadlifts - 1x20,1x15,1 x12 reps

Hamstrings

1.. Lying leg curls – 1x20,1x15,1 x12 reps

2.Standing leg curls- 1x20,1x15,1 x12 reps

Biceps

1. Incline dumbbell curls – 1x20,1x15,1 x12 reps

2.Standing pulley biceps curls- 1x20,1x15,1 x12 rep

Cardio- 20 minutes

1.Bike or treadmill

Friday

Shoulders

1. Standing side cable laterals – 1x20,1x15,1 x12 reps

2.Standing front barbell press-1x20,1x15,1 x12 reps

3. Seated bent over laterals-1x20,1x15,1 x12 reps

Triceps

1. Dip machine – 1x20,1x15,1 x12 reps

1.Close grip bench presses- 1x20,1x15 reps

2. One arm dumbbell overhead extensions – 1x20,1x15 reps

Glutes

1. Table top glute kickbacks – 1x20, 1x20, 1x20 each leg

Calves

1. Seated calf raises- 1x20,1x15,1 x12 reps

2.Standing machine calf raises- 1x20,1x15,1x12 reps

Cardio-20 minutes

1. Elliptical or bike

Saturday

Cardio

- same cardio as Tuesday

Core

-same core as Tuesday

Week 5 : Heavy week

1. Figure out your 1RM (rep max) and then go up to 90% of your 1 RM for your last set.

2. Go to failure on your last set for each exercise.

3. Rest 40-60 seconds between all sets and reps.

Sunday: Rest or 20 minute light walk

Monday: Chest+shoulders+triceps+cardio

Tuesday: Cardio+core

Wednesday: Back+hamstrings+calves

Thursday: Rest

Friday: Quads+biceps+cardio

Saturday: Cardio+core

Monday

Chest

1. Flat bar bench press - 1x10, 1x8, 1x6 reps

2. Incline bar bench press - 1x10, 1x8, 1x6 reps

3. Decline dumbbell fly - 1x10, 1x8, 1x6 reps

Shoulders

1. Dumbbell shoulder press - 1x10, 1x8, 1x6 reps

2. Dumbbell side laterals - 1x10, 1x8, 1x6 reps

3. Pulley rear delt face pulls - 1x10, 1x8, 1x6 reps

Triceps

1. Bar pulley pushdowns - 1x10, 1x8, 1x6 reps

2. Rope pulley overhead extensions - 1x10, 1x8, 1x6 reps

3. Partial mini dips - 1x10, 1x8, 1x6 reps

Cardio-25 minutes

1. Elliptical or bike

Tuesday

Cardio- 35 minutes

1. Treadmill - 10 minutes

2. Bike - 15 minutes

3. Elliptical - 10 minutes (HIIT intervals)

Core

1. Good mornings – 1x15, 1x15 reps

2. Jackknife sit ups – 1x15, 1x15, 1x15 reps

3. Side plank to reach under – 1x10, 1x10 each side

Wednesday

Back

1. Close grip low pulley row - 1x10, 1x8, 1x6 reps

2. Barbell back rows - 1x10, 1x8, 1x6 reps

3. Reverse grip pulldowns - 1x10, 1x8, 1x6 reps

4. Machine assissted chin-ups - 1x10, 1x8, 1x6 reps

Hamstrings

1. Seated leg curls - 1x10, 1x8, 1x6 reps

2. Dumbbell stiff legged deadlifts - 1x10, 1x8, 1x6 reps

Calves

1. Plate loader calf pushes - 1x10, 1x18, 1x6 reps

2. Seated calf raises - 1x10, 1x8, 1x6 reps

Friday

Quadriceps

1. Plate loader leg press - 1x10, 1x8, 1x6 reps

2. Back squats - 1x10, 1x8, 1x6 reps

3. Leg extensions - 1x10, 1x8, 1x6 reps

4. Machine leg press - 1x10, 1x8, 1x6 reps

Biceps

1. Barbell biceps curls - 1x10, 1x8, 1x6 reps

2. Incline dumbbell biceps curls - 1x10, 1x8, 1x6 reps

Cardio-25 minutes

1. Treadmile or bike

Saturday

Cardio

-same cardio as Tuesday

Core

-same core as Tuesday

Week 6: Light medium week

1. Increase weights by 2.5-5 lbs on all weights from week 4.

2. Do not go to failure on any set.

3. Rest 30-40 seconds between all sets and reps.

Sunday: Rest or 20 minute walk

Monday: Chest+back+cardio

Tuesday: Cardio+core

Wednesday: Quads+shoulders+calves

Thursday: Rest

Friday: Glutes+triceps+biceps+cardio

Saturday: Cardio+core

Monday

Chest

1. Flat dumbbell bench press - 1x15, 1x12, 1x10 reps

2. Machine chest fly - 1x15, 1x12, 1x10 reps

3. Incline dumbbell chest press - 1x15, 1x12, 1x10 reps

Back

1. Lat pulldown to front - 1x15, 1x12, 1x10 reps

2. Machine under grip pulldowns - 1x15, 1x12, 1x10 reps

3. Machine back row - 1x15, 1x12, 1x10 reps

4. T-bar rows - 1x15, 1x12, 1x10 reps

Cardio-25 minutes

1. Elliptical or bike

Tuesday

Cardio - 40 minutes

1. Rowing - 15 minutes

2. Treadmill - 15 minutes

3. Bike - 10 minutes (HIIT intervals)

Core

1. Reverse hyperextensions on stability ball - 1x15, 1x15 reps

2. Scissor kicks - 1x15, 1x15, 1x15 reps

3. Dumbbell crunches - 1x15, 1x15, 1x15 reps

4. Standing pulley twists - 1x12, 1x12 each side

Wednesday

Quadriceps

1. Bulgarian split squats - 1x15, 1x12, 1x10 for each leg

2. Leg extensions - 1x15, 1x12, 1x10, 1x10 reps

3. Standing side to side lunges - 1x12, 1x12, 1x12 for each side

Shoulders

1. Seated dumbbell side laterals - 1x15, 1x12, 1x10 reps

2. Standing front dumbbell laterals - 1x15, 1x12, 1x10 reps

3. Bent over rear cable laterals - 1x15, 1x12, 1x10 reps

Calves

1. Seated calf raises - 1x15, 1x12, 1x10 reps

2. Machine leg press calf pushes - 1x15, 1x12, 1x10 reps

Friday

Glutes

1. Standing one legged pulley glute kicks – 1x15, 1x12, 1x10 each side

Triceps

1. W-bar skull crushers - 1x15, 1x12, 1x10 reps

2. Two arm dumbbell overhead triceps extensions - 1x15, 1x12 reps

3. One arm dumbbell kickbacks - 1x15, 1x12 for each arm

Biceps

1. Standing dumbbell biceps alternate curls - 1x15, 1x12, 1x10 reps

2. Standing high pulley cable curls - 1x15, 1x12, 1x10 reps

Cardio - 25 minutes

1. Bike or treadmill

Saturday

Cardio

-same as Tuesday

Core

-same as Tuesday

Week 7: Heavy week

1. Go up 2.5-5lbs on all exercises from week 5.

2. Go to failure on your last set for each exercise.

3. Rest 40-60 seconds between all sets and reps.

Sunday: Rest or 20 minute light walk

Monday: Chest+shoulders+triceps+cardio

Tuesday: Cardio+core

Wednesday: Back+hamstrings+calves

Thursday: Rest

Friday: Quads+biceps+cardio

Saturday: Cardio+core

Monday

Chest

1. Incline bench press - 1x12, 1x10, 1x8 reps

2. Flat bench press - 1x12, 1x10, 1x8 reps

3. Decline dumbbell fly - 1x12, 1x10, 1x8 reps

Shoulders

1. Dumbbell side laterals - 1x12, 1x10, 1x8 reps

2. Dumbbell shoulder press - 1x12, 1x10, 1x8 reps

3. Pulley rear delt face pulls - 1x12, 1x10, 1x8 reps

Triceps

1. Partial mini dips - 1x12, 1x10, 1x8 reps

2. Rope pulley overhead triceps extensions - 1x12, 1x10 reps

3. Bar pulley pushdowns - 1x12, 1x10 reps

Cardio - 25 minutes

1. Treadmill or bike

Tuesday

Cardio - 40 minutes

1. Elliptical - 10 minutes

2. Bike - 20 minutes

3. Treadmill - 10 minutes (HIT)

Core

1. Superman holds - 1x20, 1x20 seconds

2. Reverse crunches - 1x15, 1x15, 1x15 reps

3. Incline sit-ups - 1x15, 1x15, 1x15 reps

4. Standing holding dumbbell side tilts - 1x12, 1x12 each side

Wednesday

Back

1. Machine assisted chin-ups - 1x12, 1x10, 1x8 reps

2. Reverse grip pulldowns - 1x12, 1x10, 1x8 reps

3. Barbell back rows - 1x12, 1x10, 1x8 reps

4. Close grip pulley rows - 1x12, 1x10, 1x8 reps

Hamstrings

1. Dumbbell stiff legged deadlifts - 1x12, 1x10, 1x8 reps

2. Seated leg curls - 1x12, 1x10, 1x8 reps

Calves

1. Seated calf raises - 1x12, 1x10, 1x8 reps

2. Plate loader calf pushes - 1x12, 1x10, 1x8 reps

Friday

Quadriceps

1. Back squats - 1x12, 1x10, 1x8 reps

2. Plate loader leg press - 1x12, 1x10, 1x8 reps

3. Machine leg press - 1x12, 1x10, 1x8 reps

4. Leg extensions - 1x12, 1x10, 1x8 reps

Biceps

1. Incline dumbbell curls - 1x12, 1x10, 1x8 reps

2. Barbell biceps curls - 1x12, 1x10, 1x8 reps

Cardio - 25 minutes

1. Elliptical or treadmill

Saturday

Cardio- 40 minutes

- same as Tuesday

Core

-same as Tuesday

Week 8: Light Medium Week

1. Keep the weights the same from week 6.

2. Do not go to failure on any set.

3. Rest 30-40 seconds between all sets and reps.

Sunday: Rest or 20 minute walk

Monday: Chest+back+cardio

Tuesday: Cardio+core

Wednesday: Quads+shoulders+calves

Thursday: Rest

Friday: Glutes+triceps+biceps+cardio

Saturday: Cardio+core

Monday

Chest

1. Incline dumbbell chest press - 1x20, 1x15, 1x10 reps

2. Machine chest fly - 1x20, 1x15, 1x10 reps

3. Flat dumbbell bench press - 1x20, 1x15, 1x10 reps

Back

1. Machine under grip pulldowns - 1x20, 1x15, 1x10 reps

2. T-bar back rows - 1x20, 1x15, 1x10 reps

3. Lat pulldown to front - 1x20, 1x15, 1x10 reps

4. Machine back row - 1x20, 1x15, 1x10 reps

Cardio - 25 minutes

1. Bike or run outside

Tuesday

Cardio-40 minutes

1. Treadmill - 20 minutes

2. Elliptical - 10 minutes

3. Rowing machine - 10 minutes (HIIT intervals)

Core

1. Single prone leg lifts - 1x15, 1x15 each side

2. Standing oblique twists with bar – 30 second x2

3. Bicycles crunches - 1x20, 1x20, 1x20 reps

Wednesday

Quadriceps

1. Leg extensions - 1x20, 1x15, 1x12, 1x10 reps

2. Bulgarian spilt squats - 1x15, 1x12, 1x10 each side

3. Standing side to side lunges - 1x15, 1x15, 1x15 each side

Shoulders

1. Front dumbbell laterals - 1x20, 1x15, 1x10 reps

2. Side dumbbell laterals - 1x20, 1x15, 1x10 reps

3. Bent over rear laterals - 1x20, 1x15, 1x10 reps

Calves

1. Machine leg calf pushes - 1x20, 1x15, 1x10 reps

2. Seated calf raises - 1x20, 1x15, 1x10 reps

Friday

Glutes

1. Standing one legged pulley glute kicks – 1x20, 1x15, 1x12 each side

Triceps

1. W-bar skull crushers - 1x20, 1x15, 1x10 reps

2. One arm dumbbell triceps kickbacks - 1x20, 1x15 reps

3. Two arm dumbbell overhead triceps extensions - 1x20, 1x15 reps

Biceps

1. Standing dumbbell alternate curls - 1x20, 1x15, 1x10 reps

2. Standing high pulley cable curls - 1x20, 1x15, 1x10 reps

Cardio-25 minutes

1. Treadmill

Saturday

Cardio

-same as Tuesday

Core

-same as Tuesday

SECTION B – BULK UP AND GAIN MUSCLE

EATING FOR MUSCULAR GAINS

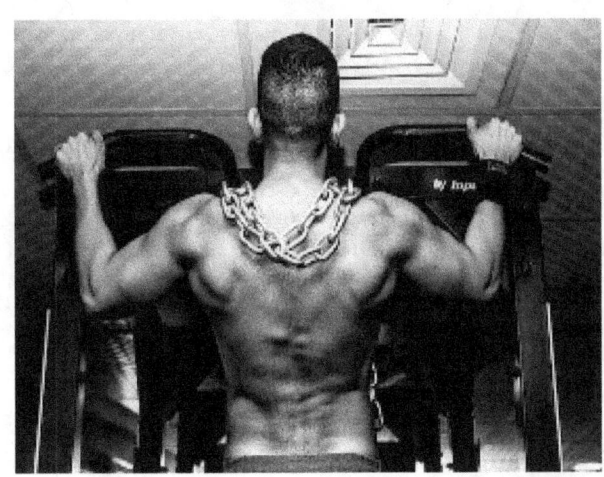

Most superheroes are known for their super powers and bulging muscles, such as Superman when he picks up a truck. His muscles ripple as he exerts force.

Muscle basically translates to physical power and strength. People work out to feel healthier, stronger, and to live a longer life. As we have learned before, our muscle mass declines as we age. A person who carries more muscle mass will burn more calories at rest verses a person with average muscle mass. Most men and even some women who weight train want to look physically powerful.

Now we come to the fun part, bulking up. Dieting is not a fun process, but the end result makes it worth while. I love to eat because food taste so damn good. Who doesn't like to sink their teeth into a nice juicy burger. Guess what, you can eat a burger while bulking up and not feel guilty. Gaining muscle requires an excess amount of calories.

Did you know around 3500 calories equals to one pound of body weight? Going back to the male who is 35 and has a REE of 1657 kcal per day. The BMR and REE can be used as a base for muscle gain and fat loss. Once a person has established their REE, it is crucial they stay in the positive energy balance to gain weight.

Next is to look at the person's physical activity output. Weight training sessions can burn up 200-300 calories per session depending on the intensity level. So 2-3 weight training sessions a week would be an extra 600-900 extra calories on top of the 1657. That would bring the caloric intake up between 2257 and 2557 calories. I would then add an extra 300-400 calories to be in the positive energy balance making total caloric intake between 2657 and 2957. In order to gain muscle naturally a person must gain some body fat also.

Some experts say 1 pound of muscle for every 2-3 lbs of fat but everyone is different so there is no exact number. It is impossible to gain pure muscle mass unless the person is chemically enhanced. Chemically enhanced means the use steroids, growth hormone, clenburatol, and a list of other various drugs.

In order to lose body fat a person must follow a diet of clean eating and caloric reduction. One example of clean protein source would be a grilled chicken breast with lemon, salt, and garlic. A bad choice would be deep-fried chicken or deep-fried, battered fish. In order to gain muscle a person must follow a higher caloric diet, so eating a cheat meal more frequently is not a bad idea. When losing body fat, it is crucial to eat clean 80-90 percent of the time but when gaining muscle a person can cheat more frequently since their calories are not as restrictive.

One of the most talked about issues when trying to add muscle mass is the protein intake and what is the proper amount. As I said before someone who is active should consume between 1.6 to 2.2 grams per kilo/day. So a person who weighs 75 kg would consume between 120-165 grams per day. If a person were to eat 3 small meals and 3 snacks a day, this would work out roughly to 20-27.5 grams of protein per meal. Using these numbers as a guide, I would round it up to 30 grams per meal.

When building muscle, it is important to also eat enough carbohydrates and fats. If a good ratio to follow is 30% protein, 50% carbohydrates, and 20% fat. If you find you're gaining too much fat, you can cut back on the carbs by 10% and increase the ratio of protein by 10%. A person eating 3000 calories a day at 30/50/20 would have the following ratio breakdowns. Protein breakdown would be 900 (3000x.30) calories and would be 225 (900/4) grams per day. The person would consume 37.5 grams per meal if they were to eat 6 times in a day. Carbohydrates would be 1500 (3000x.5) calories and would be 375 (1500/4) grams per day. The person would eat 62.5 (375/4) grams per meal if they were to eat 6 times in a day. Fats would be 600 (3000x.2) calories and would be 67 (600/9) grams per day. The person would consume 11 (67/9) grams per meal if they were to eat 6 times in a day.

After a person weight trains, it is best they consume some post-workout food or a post-workout shake. I always have a protein and carbohydrate shake after I weight train. The shake consists of 60-80 grams of carbohydrates and 40-50 grams of protein.

When a person weight trains they rip the muscle and use up their stored glycogen inside of the muscle. So the carbohydrates are used to replenish the lost glycogen and the protein is used to repair the muscle. It is best to have a shake or meal within 30-40 minutes after training.

The last thing a person wants is to let the body starve and turn on itself for the missing nutrients. A post-workout shake for males should consist of 50-60 grams of carbs after and 40-50 grams of protein after.

A post-workout shake for females should consist of 20-30 grams of carbs and 20-30 grams of protein after. To keep things simple, any protein powder works and any fast-acting carbohydrates that is high on the GI charts.

Carbohydrates like white rice, instant oatmeal, cornflakes, and sugars. If a person where to choose a protein food source, they should stick to faster digesting proteins like chicken, turkey, and fish.

These are just guidelines to follow but the main point to is keep a positive energy intake when trying to build muscle mass. If you are unsure of what to eat go back and read the protein, fat, and carbohydrate chapters over again.

If you are starting to look like a good year blimp from all the extra calories add some cardiovascular workouts to your schedule or change the protein and carbohydrate ratio. There is no real secret to gaining muscle but being consistent with your eating, sleeping, and training.

TOP 6 RULES FOR GAINING MUSCLE

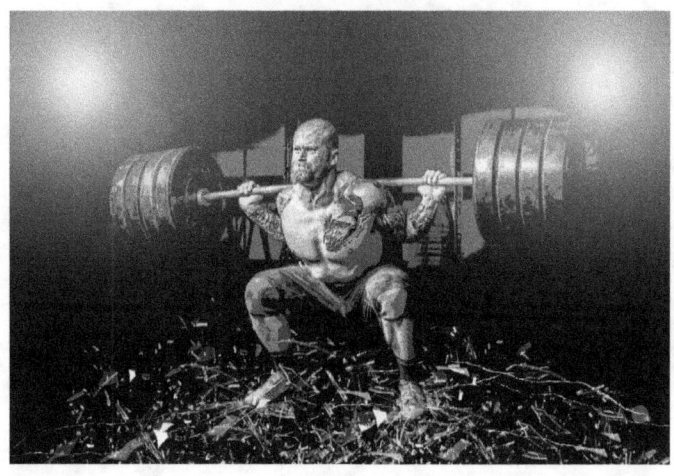

1. Never let yourself get hungry. You need a consistent flow of nutrients to your muscles all the time when building muscle. Have snacks around you all the time. Snacks like protein bars, nuts, and cheese.

2. Train heavy or increase the volume of force on your muscles. Your muscles grow from extra stress that comes from heavier weight or increased volume.

3. Get adequate rest in between your workouts and at night. Your muscles grow when you rest. Do not over train as this is counter productive to growth. If you have not fully recovered from your previous workout, take another day off. More is not always better.

4. Do not stop cardiovascular workouts completely. When people bulk up, they often neglect cardio. Just cut down on the volume and intensity of those types of workouts. Just do light walking instead of running. Doing light cardio will help with keeping your BMR up, which will help burn more calories efficiently.

5. The top 5 supplements to use when bulking are creatine hydrochloride (HCL), weight gainers, glutamine, vitamins(if needed), and whey or isolate protein powder.

6. Stay hydrated all the time. Your body functions best when fully hydrated. If your system is firing on all cylinders, you will create a more anabolic effect for muscle growth. Aim for 8-12 glasses of water or more a day.

TWO DIET EXAMPLES OF EATING PLANS FOR GAINING MUSCLE

EATING PLAN 1

This is an example of a diet for a male who does not have as much time to eat, slower metabolism, but still wants to gain muscle mass.

He would eat 3 meals and 2 snacks. Please see next page.

Meal 1 8:00am	2 slices whole grain toast with 2 tsp. natural peanut butter 2 whole eggs with ketchup and cheese 1 cup of carrots 1 medium pear
Meal 2 12:00pm	7-8oz salmon with lemon, garlic, brown sugar 2 cups of Caesar salad 1 large potato with cheese and butter
Snack 1 3:00pm	2 promax or quest protein bars
Meal 3 6:00pm	7-8oz steak with steak sauce 2 cups pasta with spaghetti sauce 2 cups kale and lettuce with Italian salad dressing
Snack 2 8:30pm	5-6 oz protein source 1 cup of fruit yogurt or 2 cups of cottage cheese

EATING PLAN 2

This is a variation for a female who would want to gain some muscle or who has a fast metabolism and needs to put on some body weight.

Most females want to lose weight but there are some who have an extremely fast metabolism and gaining muscle is quite a challenge.

I have trained over a few hundred females so I have come across every type of body and metabolism type. Please see next page.

Meal 1 8:00am	whole egg with 1 egg white and cheese 1 slice of whole grain toast tsp. natural peanut butter or jam 1/2 cup of grapes
Meal 2 12:00pm	3-4oz chicken with barbecue sauce 1 cup steamed broccoli 1 cup brown rice with soya sauce
Snack 1 3:00pm	1 scoop whey isolate 1 cup fruit yogurt
Meal 3 6:00pm	3-4oz lean ground turkey with curry sauce 1.5 cup of mixed salad with Greek dressing 1/2 yam or small baked potato with cheese and butter
Snack 2 8:30pm	1/2 avocado 2-3oz fish or 1/2 cup unsalted nuts 1 cup fruit yogurt

5 HIGH CALORIE PROTEIN SHAKES

In the quest to build muscle mass taking in those extra calories is important for recovery and growth.

When you are eating over 4000 calories, high calorie protein shakes are a good option.

Here are 5 high calorie protein shakes to incorporate into your bulking diet.

High Protein Milkshake

1 cup whole milk
1 scoop whey protein powder
1/4 cup dry milk powder
3/4 cup ice cream

Add ice cream, protein powder, and milk powder to milk and beat well.

Calories = 533

Protein= 36

Strawberry Yogurt Frost

1 envelope strawberry instant breakfast
1 scoop whey protein powder
1 cup whole milk
1/4 cup dry milk powder
1/3 cup strawberry yogurt
6 ice cubes

Combine all ingredients in a blender. Blend until smooth.

Calories = 524

Protein = 41

OJ and Cinnamon Smoothie

1 envelope vanilla instant breakfast

1 scoop whey protein powder

1 cup whole milk

1/4 cup dry milk powder

3 Tbs thawed orange juice concentrate

1/8 tsp ground cinnamon

6 ice cubes

Combine all ingredients in a blender. Blend until smooth.

Calories = 537

Protein = 38

Mocha-Banana Shake

1 envelope chocolate instant breakfast

1 scoop whey protein powder

1 cup whole milk

1/4 cup dry milk powder

1 medium ripe banana

1/2 tsp instant coffee crystals

Combine all ingredients in a blender. Blend until smooth.

Calories = 542

Protein = 39

Hawaiian Slush

6 oz. Hawaiian Punch

1 scoop whey protein powder

1/3 cup dry milk powder

1/2 cup lemon sherbet

1 Tbs sugar

3 ice cubes

Combine all ingredients in a blender and blend for about 10 seconds. Fruit juice can be used in place of the Hawaiian Punch.

Calories = 415

Protein = 28

WHAT ARE YOUR GOALS

What are your goals?

Do you want to gain 5 lbs, 10lbs, or bench press your body weight?

Write down some of your goals below.

Remember to be realistic as building muscle takes time. If you set 3 small goals to gain 5 lbs, that equates to an overall gain of 15lbs.

1.

2.

3.

TRAINING GUIDELINES

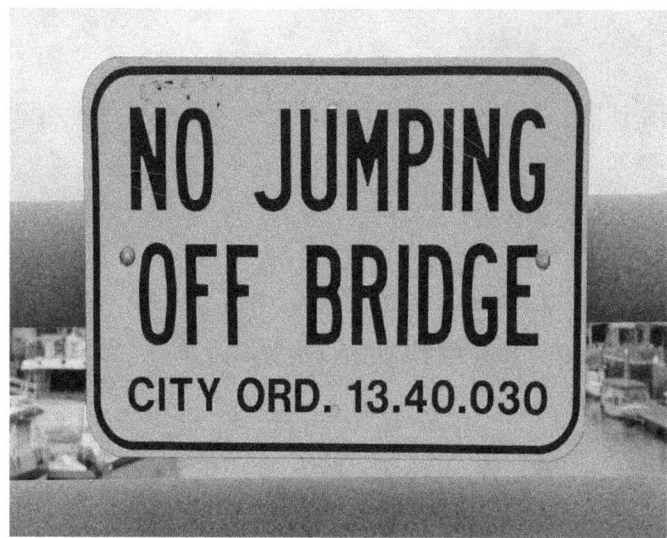

Read and memorize this before you start your training program. These are the same training guidelines for the fat loss section. I decided to include them again just in case you are just going to do the bulk up phase.

1. Always practice good form. A good controlled set will recruit more muscle fibers verses throwing the weights around.

2. Do one warm up set with a lighter weight. This will allow you to practice the exercise and execute good form for the next sets.

3. Lower the weight in a controlled manner. The lowering part of the rep is called the negative (eccentric) portion. More control in the lowering portion will recruit more muscle fibers.

4. Breathe out with force. Never hold your breath during a set. Your muscles need oxygen to keep working and to expel carbon dioxide. A red face does not look attractive.

5. Know when to stop. Sometimes it is not good to push beyond failure. Pushing yourself to hard all the time can lead to injuries.

6. Record your weights in a book to track your progress. This is how to track your progress. In the paperback edition, you will be able to write the weight right beside the exercise.

7. Do large muscle groups before smaller muscle groups as they require the most energy. Doing biceps before training your back is detrimental to your back workout as your arms will fatigue first.

8. Always set goals before you start any training program. This will give you more purpose and will help you reach your goal.

9. Try not to grunt or scream when you do your set or reps. Save your energy for the next set. You are not impressing anyone.

10. If you are unsure of any exercises just look them up in the internet. Study the form of every exercise.

11. Weigh yourself once a week at the same time and day. Preferably in the morning before you eat breakfast.

TWO WEEK BEGINNER TRAINING PROGRAM

Are you a beginner and have no training experience?

If you answered yes, just follow this two week program as a warm up. Learn all the exercises and then proceed to the eight week training program after.

This is the same program in the lose weight and get ripped section. I decided to include them again just in case you are just going to do the bulk up phase.

Week 1

Sunday: Rest

Monday: Workout 1 (full body workout)

Tuesday: Rest

Wednesday: Cardio + core (abs)

Thursday: Workout 2 (full body workout)

Friday: Rest

Saturday: Light cardio

Monday

Workout 1

1. Warm up for 5-6 minutes on a cardio machine

2. Lat pull down to front – 1x12, 1x10, 1x8 reps

3. Machine leg press – 1x12, 1x10, 1x8 reps

4. Machine back row – 1x12, 1x10, 1x8 reps

5. Machine bench press – 1x12, 1x10, 1x8 reps

6. Lying prone machine hamstring curls – 1x12, 1x10, 1x8 reps

7. Machine shoulder press – 1x12, 1x10, 1x8 reps

8. Seated adductor machine – 1x15, 1x12, 1x10 reps

9. Cool down for 5-6 minutes on a cardio machine

10. Static stretching or use my stretching app

https://goo.gl/RLSCHo

Wednesday

Cardio – 20 minutes

1. Bike – 10 minutes

2. Treadmill – 10 minutes

Core

1. Bird dogs - 1 x12, 1x12 reps

2. Seated leg lifts – 1x15, 1x15 for each side

3. Cable crunches - 1x15, 1x15 reps

4. Standing medicine ball twists – 1 minute

Thursday

Workout 2

1. Warm up for 5-6 minutes on a cardio machine

2. Reverse grip bar pull downs – 1x15, 1x12, 1x10 reps

3. Seated machine leg extensions – 1x15, 1x12, 1x10 reps

4. Pulley low grip back rows – 1x15, 1x12, 1x10 reps

5. Flat dumbbell chest fly – 1x15, 1x12, 1x10 reps

6. Seated upright hamstring curls – 1x15, 1x12, 1x10 reps

7. Dumbbell side laterals – 1x15, 1x12, 1x10 reps

8. Seal jacks – 1x15, 1x15 reps

9. Machine triceps extension – 1x15, 1x12, 1x10 reps

10. Machine biceps curls – 1x15, 1x10 reps

11. Cool down for 5-6 minutes on a cardio machine

12. Static stretching or use my stretching app

https://goo.gl/RLSCHo

Saturday

Cardio – 20 minutes

1. Elliptical – 10 minutes

2. Rowing – 10 minutes

Core

1. Hold superman – 1x15, 1x15 seconds

2. Standing bicycle crunches – 1x15, 1x15 reps

3. Oblique cable twists – 1x15, 1x15 each side

Week 2

Sunday: Rest or walking for 20 minutes

Monday: Workout 1 (same as week 1)

Tuesday: Rest

Wednesday: Cardio + core (same workout as week 1)

Thursday: Workout 2 (same as week 1)

Friday: Rest

Saturday: Cardio + core (same workout as week 1)

EIGHT WEEK STRENGTH TRAINING PROGRAM FOR MEN

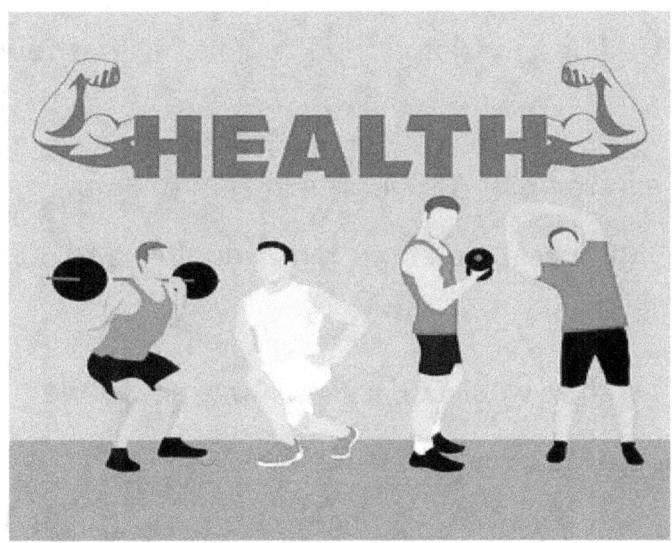

If you have completed the two week beginner program, you are now ready for the eight week training program.

If you are not a beginner, just jump into this training program. If your level 2, add an extra set to each exercise to suit your needs.

Get ready to grow and train!

8 Week Strength & Mass Building Program For Men – Level 1

Week 1: Heavy week

1. Figure out your 1RM (rep max) and then go up to 90% of your 1RM on your last set.

- a 200 lb bench press would be 180 for the last set of 4 reps

2. Figure out your BMR (basal metabolic rate) and then add 500-600 calories extra per day.

- total caloric intake for the week 500 x 7 = 3500 extra calories

- another easier method is to use your TDEE

3. Always do a 5-8 minute warm-up and 5-8 minute cool down before and after every training session.

This should include static stretching after each exercise session.

4. Use ascending pyramiding for all set and exercises throughout this program.

5. If you are unsure of any exercise just look it up on the internet.

6. Rest 30-60 seconds in between all sets and reps.

7. Go to failure on the last set and record all your weights.

Sunday: Cardio 20-25 minutes + core

Monday: Back + hamstrings

Tuesday: Chest + triceps

Wednesday: Rest day

Thursday: Shoulders + biceps + forearms + core

Friday: Quadriceps + calves + traps

Saturday: Rest day

Sunday

Cardio

1. Bike or tread mile - 20-25 minutes

Core

1. Hold Superman - 1 x 15, 1x15 seconds

2. Scissor kicks – 1x15, 1x15, 1x15 reps

3. Dumbbell crunches – 1x15, 1x15, 1x15 reps

4. Side planks - 1 x 15 seconds each side

Monday

Back

1. Deadlifts - 1x10, 1x8, 1x6 reps

2. Reverse grip pull downs - 1x10, 1x8, 1x6 reps

3. Barbell back rows - 1x10, 1x8, 1x6 reps

4. Pulley seated back rows - 1x10, 1x8, 1x6 reps

Hamstrings

1. Lying leg curls - 1x10, 1x8, 1x6 reps

2. Stiff legged dead lifts - 1x10, 1x8, 1x6 reps

Tuesday

Chest

1. Incline bench press - 1x10, 1x8, 1x6 reps

2. Flat bench press - 1x10, 1x8, 1x6 reps

3. Dumbbell pullovers - 1x10, 1x8, 1x6 reps

Triceps

1. Bar pulley push downs - 1x10, 1x8, 1x6 reps

2. Pulley rope overhead extensions - 1x10, 1x8 reps

3. W-bar skull crushers - 1x10, 1x8 reps

Thursday

Shoulders

1. Seated barbell front press - 1x10, 1x8, 1x6 reps

2. Dumbbell side laterals - 1x10, 1x8, 1x6 reps

3. Bent over dumbbell rear laterals - 1x10, 1x8, 1x6 reps

Biceps

1. Barbell biceps curls - 1x10, 1x8, 1x6 reps

2. Seated machine biceps curls - 1x10, 1x8, 1x6 reps

Forearms

1. Behind the body bar curls - 1x10, 1x8 reps

2. Standing reverse bar curls - 1x10, 1x8 reps

Core

1. Same core as Sunday workout

Friday

Quadriceps

1. Plate loader leg press - 1x10, 1x8, 1x6, 1x4 reps

2. Back squats - 1x10, 1x8, 1x6, 1x4 reps

3. Leg extensions - 1x10, 1x8, 1x6, 1x4 reps

Calves

1. Seated calf raises - 1x12, 1x10, 1x8 reps

2. Standing calf raises - 1x12, 1x10, 1x8 reps

Traps

Dumbbell shrugs - 1x10, 1x8, 1x6 reps

Week 2: Medium Light Week

1. Go up to 70% 1RM

- a 200 lb bench press would be 140 for 8 reps on the last set

2. Do not go to failure on any set

Sunday: Cardio 20-25 minutes + core

Monday: Chest + back

Tuesday: Shoulders + hamstrings

Wednesday: Rest

Thursday: Quadriceps + adductors + abductors + calves + traps

Friday: Triceps + biceps + forearms + core

Sat: Rest

Sunday

Cardio

1. Tread mile or elliptical - 20-25 minutes

Core

1. Back extensions on the mat – 1x15, 1x15 reps

2. Reverse crunches – 1x12, 1x12, 1x12 reps

3. Cable crunches – 1x12, 1x12, 1x12 reps

4. Dumbbell side tilts - 1x15 each side

Monday

Chest

1. Regular pushups - 1x15, 1x15, 1x15 reps

2. Incline dumbbell chest press - 1x15, 1x12, 1x10 reps

3. Cable crossovers - 1x15, 1x12, 1x10 reps

Back

1. Seated machine back row - 1x15, 1x12, 1x10 reps

2. Close grip pull down - 1x15, 1x12, 1x10 reps

3. One arm dumbbell back rows - 1x15, 1x12, 1x10 reps

4. High pulley pullovers - 1x15, 1x12, 1x10 reps

Tuesday

Shoulders

1. Machine shoulder press - 1x15, 1x12, 1x10 reps

2. Barbell upright rows - 1x15, 1x12, 1x10 reps

3. Pulley face pulls - 1x15, 1x12, 1x10 reps

Hamstrings

1. Seated hamstring curls - 1x15, 1x12, 1x10 reps

2. Dumbbell dead lifts - 1x15, 1x12, 1x10 reps

Thursday

Quadriceps/abductors/adductors

1. Leg extensions - 1x15, 1x12, 1x10 reps

2. Plie dumbbell squats - 1x15, 1x12, 1x10 reps

3. Seated adductor machine - 1x15, 1x12 reps

4. Seated abductor machine - 1x15, 1x12 reps

5. Bulgarian split squats - 1x15, 1x12, 1x10 for each leg

Calves

1. One legged standing dumbbell calf raises - 1x15, 1x12, 1x10 for each side

2. Seated calf raises - 1x15, 1x12, 1x10 reps

Traps

1. Barbell shrugs - 1x15, 1x12, 1x10 reps

Friday

Triceps

1. Close grip bench presses - 1x15, 1x12, 1x10 reps

2. One arm overhead dumbbell triceps extension - 1x15, 1x12 each side

3. One arm dumbbell triceps kickbacks - 1x15, 1x12 each side

Biceps

1. Alternate dumbbell bicep curls - 1x15, 1x12, 1x10 reps

2. Preacher curls - 1x15, 1x12, 1x10 reps

Forearms

1. Reverse preacher curls - 1x15, 1x12 reps

2. Seated dumbbell palms up wrist curls - 1x15, 1x12 reps

Core

1. Same core as Sunday

Week 3: Heavy Week

1. Go up 5-10 lbs from week 1 on all exercises

2. A 5 lb increase on smaller muscle groups and a 10 lb increase on larger muscle groups

3. Go to failure on the last set

Sunday: Cardio 20-25 minutes + core

Monday: Back + hamstrings

Tuesday: Chest + triceps

Wed: Rest

Thursday: Shoulders + biceps + forearms + core

Friday: Quadriceps + calves + traps

Saturday: Rest

Sunday

Cardio

1. Tread mile or rowing machine - 20-25 minutes

Core

1. Single prone leg lifts - 1x12, 1x12 each leg

2. Bicycles - 1x15, 1x15, 1x15 reps

3. Side plank reaches - 1x10 each side

Monday

Back

1. Barbell back rows - 1x12, 1x10, 1x8 reps

2. Reverse grip pull downs - 1x12, 1x10, 1x8 reps

3. Bar deadlifts - 1x12, 1x10, 1x8 reps

4. Chin ups - 1x12, 1x10, 1x8 reps (use chin up assisted machine)

Hamstrings

1. Lying leg curls - 1x12, 1x10, 1x8 reps

2. Seated leg curls - 1x12, 1x10, 1x8 reps

Tuesday

Chest

1. Flat bench press - 1x12, 1x10, 1x8 reps

2. Incline bench press - 1x12, 1x10, 1x8 reps

3. Incline dumbbell fly - 1x12, 1x10, 1x8 reps

Triceps

1. Bar skull crushers - 1x12, 1x10, 1x8 reps

2. Pulley push downs - 1x12, 1x10 reps

3. Pulley rope triceps overhead extensions - 1x12, 1x10 reps

Thursday

Shoulders

1. Dumbbell side laterals - 1x12, 1x10, 1x8 reps

2. Seated barbell front shoulder press - 1x12, 1x10, 1x8 reps

3. Bent over dumbbell rear laterals raises- 1x12, 1x10, 1x8 reps

Biceps

1. Seated machine biceps curls - 1x12, 1x10, 1x8 reps

2. Barbell biceps curls - 1x12, 1x10, 1x8 reps

Forearms

1. Standing reverse curls - 1x12, 1x10 reps

2. Behind the body curls - 1x12, 1x10 reps

Core

1. Same workout as Sunday

Friday

Quadriceps

1. Back squats - 1x12, 1x10, 1x8 reps

2. Leg press - 1x12, 1x10, 1x8 reps

3. Leg extensions - 1x12, 1x10, 1x8 reps

4. Hack squats - 1x12, 1x10, 1x8 reps

Calves

1. Standing calf raises - 1x12, 1x10, 1x8 reps

2. Seated calf raises - 1x12, 1x10, 1x8 reps

Traps

Dumbbell shrugs - 1x12, 1x10, 1x8 reps

Week 4: Medium - Light week

1. Keep the same weights as week 2

2. We are increasing the resistance by increasing the reps

3. Do not go to failure for any sets

Sunday: Cardio 20-25 minutes + core

Monday: Chest + back

Tuesday: Shoulders + hamstrings

Wednesday: Rest

Thursday: Quadriceps + adductors + abductors + traps + calves

Friday: Triceps + biceps + forearms + core

Saturday: Rest

Sunday

Cardio

1. Treadmill or elliptical - 20-25 minutes

Core

1. Bird dogs - 1x15, 1x15 reps

2. Dumbbell side tilts - 1x15 each side

3. Stability ball passes - 1x10, 1x10, 1x10 reps

Monday

Back

1. Close grip V-bar pull down - 1x20, 1x15, 1x12 reps

2. Machine back row - 1x20, 1x15, 1x12 reps

3. High pulley pullovers - 1x20, 1x15, 1x12 reps

4. One arm dumbbell rows - 1x20, 1x15, 1x12 reps

Chest

1. Incline dumbbell chest press - 1x20, 1x15, 1x12 reps

2. Regular pushups - 1x15, 1x15, 1x15 reps

3. Cable crossovers - 1x20, 1x15, 1x12 reps

Tuesday

Shoulders

1. Machine shoulder press - 1x20, 1x15, 1x12 reps

2. Pulley face pulls - 1x20, 1x15, 1x12 reps

3. Barbell upright rows - 1x20, 1x15, 1x12 reps

Hamstrings

1. Dumbbell stiff legged dead lifts - 1x20, 1x15, 1x12 reps

2. Seated hamstring curls - 1x20, 1x15, 1x12 reps

Thursday

Quadriceps/adductors/abductors

1. Leg extensions - 1x20, 1x15, 1x12 reps

2. Bulgarian split squats - 1x20, 1x15, 1x12 for each leg

3. Seated adductor machine - 1x20, 1x15 reps

4. Seated abductor machine - 1x20, 1x15 reps

5. Plie dumbbell squats - 1x20, 1x15, 1x12 reps

Calves

1. Seated calf raises - 1x20, 1x15, 1x12 reps

2. One legged standing dumbbell calf raises - 1x20, 1x15, 1x12 for each side

Traps

1. Barbell shrugs - 1x20, 1x15, 1x12 reps

Friday

Triceps

1. Seated overhead dumbbell triceps extensions - 1x20, 1x15, 1x12 reps

2. Close grip bench presses - 1x20, 1x15 reps

3. One arm dumbbell kickbacks - 1x20, 1x15 reps

Biceps

1. Preacher bar bicep curls - 1x20, 1x15, 1x10 reps

2. Alternate dumbbell biceps curls - 1x20, 1x15, 1x10 reps

Forearms

1. Seated palms up wrist curls - 1x20, 1x15 reps

2. Reverse preacher curls - 1x20, 1x15 reps

Core

1. Same workout as Sunday

Week 5: Heavy Week

1. Figure out your 1RM

2. Go to up to 90% of your 1RM for all exercises.

3. Go to failure for the last set.

Sunday: Cardio 20-25 minutes + core

Monday: Chest + triceps

Tuesday: Back + biceps

Wednesday: Rest

Thursday: Shoulders + traps + forearms + core

Friday: Quadriceps +hamstrings+ calves

Saturday: Rest

Sunday

Cardio

1. Elliptical or Rower - 20-25 minutes

Core

1. Hold superman – 1x15, 1x15 seconds

2. Dumbbell crunches – 1x15, 1x15, 1x15 reps

3. Scissor kicks – 1x15, 1x15, 1x15 reps

4. Side planks – 1x15 seconds each side

Monday

Chest

1. Flat dumbbell bench press - 1x10, 1x8, 1x6 reps

2. Machine chest fly - 1x10, 1x8, 1x6 reps

3. Incline dumbbell bench press - 1x10, 1x8, 1x6 reps

Triceps

1. Rope triceps push downs - 1x10, 1x8, 1x6 reps

2. Decline dumbbell triceps extensions - 1x10, 1x8 reps

3. Mini-dips - 1x10, 1x8 reps

Tuesday

Back

1. Close grip v-bar pull downs - 1x10, 1x8, 1x6 reps

2. Seated v-bar back pulley rows - 1x10, 1x8, 1x6 reps

3. Under grip chin ups - 1x10, 1x8, 1x6 reps

4. One arm dumbbell back rows - 1x10, 1x8, 1x6 reps

Biceps

1. Machine biceps curls - 1x10, 1x8, 1x6 reps

2. Incline dumbbell biceps curls - 1x10, 1x8, 1x6 reps

Thursday

Shoulders

1. Seated dumbbell shoulder presses - 1x10, 1x8, 1x6 reps

2. Cable side laterals - 1x10, 1x8, 1x6 reps

3. Machine rear delt fly - 1x10, 1x8, 1x6 reps

Traps

1. Barbell shrugs - 1x10, 1x8, 1x6 reps

Forearms

1. Dumbbell hammer curls - 1x10, 1x8, 1x6 reps

2. Behind the body curls - 1x10, 1x8, 1x6 reps

Core

1. Same as Sunday

Friday

Quadriceps

1. Back squats - 1x10, 1x8, 1x6 reps

2. Leg extensions - 1x10, 1x8, 1x6 reps

3. Machine leg press - 1x10, 1x8, 1x6 reps

4. Single leg extensions - 1x10, 1x8, 1x6 reps

Hamstrings

1. Standing leg curls - 1x10, 1x8 1x6 reps

2. Lying leg curls - 1x10, 1x8, 1x6 reps

Calves

1. Leg press machine calf pushes - 1x12, 1x10, 1x8 reps

2. Seated calf raises - 1x12, 1x10, 1x8 reps

Week 6: Medium Light Week

1. Go up 5 lbs for small muscle groups from week 4

2. Go up 10 lbs for larger muscle groups from week 4

3. Do not go to failure on any set

Sunday: Cardio 20-25 minutes + core

Monday: Chest + quadriceps

Tuesday: Shoulders + triceps

Wednesday: Rest

Thursday: Back + hamstrings

Friday: Traps + biceps + forearms + core

Saturday: Rest

Sunday

Cardio

1. Tread mile or bike - 20-25 minutes

Core

1. On stomach back extensions - 1x15, 1x15 reps

2. Cable crunches - 1x15, 1x15, 1x15 reps

3. Reverse crunches - 1x15, 1x15, 1x15 reps

4. Dumbbell side tilts - 1x15, 1x15 each side

Monday

Chest

1. Incline dumbbell flye - 1x15, 1x12, 1x10 reps

2. Flat machine bench press - 1x15, 1x12, 1x10 reps

3. Machine chest fly - 1x15, 1x12, 1x10 reps

Quadriceps

1. Holding dumbbell squats - 1x15, 1x12, 1x10 reps

2. Leg extensions - 1x15, 1x12, 1x10 reps

3. Side lunges on bosu - 1x15, 1x15, 1x15 for each side

4. Hack squats - 1x15, 1x12, 1x10 reps

Tuesday

Shoulders

1. Dumbbell front laterals - 1x15, 1x12, 1x10 reps

2. Dumbbell side laterals - 1x15, 1x12, 1x10 reps

3. Dumbbell rear laterals - 1x15, 1x12, 1x10 reps

Triceps

1. W-bar skull crushers - 1x15, 1x12, 1x10 reps

2. Rope pulley overhead triceps extensions - 1x15, 1x12 reps

3. Triceps dip machine - 1x15, 1x12 reps

Thursday

Back

1. T-bar rows - 1x15, 1x12, 1x10 reps

2. Seated back pulley rows - 1x15, 1x12, 1x10 reps

3. Pull down to front - 1x15, 1x12, 1x10 reps

4. Under grip pull downs - 1x15, 1x12, 1x10 reps

Hamstrings

1. Supine one legged ball curls - 1x10, 1x10, 1x10 for each leg

2. Dumbbell stiff legged dead lifts - 1x15, 1x12, 1x10 reps

Calves

1. Seated calf raises - 1x15, 1x12, 1x10 reps

2. Plate loader leg press calf pushes - 1x15, 1x12, 1x10 reps

Friday

Traps

1. Dumbbell shrugs - 1x15, 1x12, 1x10, 1x8 reps

Biceps

1. Bar pulley biceps curls - 1x15, 1x12, 1x10 reps

2. Pulley overhead cable curls - 1x15, 1x12, 1x10 reps

Forearms

1. Reverse barbell curls - 1x15, 1x12 reps

2. Cross the bench bar flexor curls - 1x15, 1x12 reps

Core

1. Same as Sunday workout

Week 7: Heavy Week

1. Go up 5lbs for smaller muscle groups from week 5

2. Go up 10 lbs for larger muscle groups from week 5

3. Go to failure for the last set

Sunday: Cardio + core

Monday: Chest + triceps

Tuesday: Back + biceps

Wednesday: Rest

Thursday: Shoulders + traps + forearms + core

Friday: Quadriceps + hamstrings + calves

Saturday: Rest

Sunday

Cardio

1. Rower or Tread mile - 20-25 minutes

Core

1. Single prone leg lifts - 1x15, 1x15 each leg

2. Elbow plank - 30 seconds x2

3. V-sit holds – 30 seconds x2

4. Standing medicine ball twists - 1 minute

Monday

Chest

1. Incline dumbbell chest press - 1x12, 1x10, 1x8 reps

2. Machine chest fly - 1x12, 1x10, 1x8 reps

3. Flat dumbbell bench press - 1x12, 1x10, 1x8 reps

Triceps

1. Rope triceps push downs - 1x12, 1x10, 1x8 reps

2. Partial mini- dips - 1x12, 1x10 reps

3. Decline dumbbell triceps extensions - 1x12, 1x10 reps

Tuesday

Back

1. Close grip V-bar pull down - 1x12, 1x10, 1x8 reps

2. One arm back dumbbell rows - 1x12, 1x10, 1x8 reps

3. Under grip chin ups - 1x12, 1x10, 1x8 reps

4. Seated V-bar back pulley rows - 1x12, 1x10, 1x8 reps

Biceps

1. Incline dumbbell curls - 1x12, 1x10, 1x8 reps

2. Machine biceps curls - 1x12, 1x10, 1x8 reps

Thursday

Shoulders

1. Cable side laterals - 1x12, 1x10, 1x8 reps

2. Dumbbell shoulder presses - 1x12, 1x10, 1x8 reps

3. Machine rear delt fly - 1x12, 1x10, 1x8 reps

Traps

1. Barbell shrugs - 1x12, 1x10, 1x8 reps

Forearms

1. Behind the body bar curls - 1x12, 1x10 reps

2. Dumbbell hammer curls - 1x12, 1x10 reps

Core

1. Same workout as Sunday

Friday

Quadriceps

1. Machine leg press - 1x12, 1x10, 1x8 reps

2. Leg extensions - 1x12, 1x10, 1x8 reps

3. Back squats - 1x12, 1x10, 1x8 reps

4. Single leg extensions - 1x12, 1x10 reps

Hamstrings

1. Lying leg curls - 1x12, 1x10, 1x8 reps

2. Standing leg curls, 1x12, 1x10, 1x18 reps

Calves

1. Seated calf raises - 1x12, 1x10, 1x8 reps

2. Leg press calf pushes - 1x12, 1x10, 1x8 reps

Week 8: Light Medium Week

1. Use same weights as week 6 and we will increase resistance by reps

2. Do not go to failure any set

Sunday: Cardio + core

Monday: Chest + quadriceps

Tuesday: Shoulders + triceps

Wednesday: Rest

Thursday: Back + hamstrings + calves

Friday: Traps + biceps + forearms + core

Saturday: Rest

Sunday

Cardio

1. Bike or tread mile - 20-25 minutes

Core

1. Land swimming – 1x15, 1x15 seconds

2. Stability ball pikes – 1x15, 1x15, 1x15 reps

3. Standing oblique bar twists - 1x1 minute

Monday

1. Flat machine bench press - 1x20, 1x15, 1x12 reps

2. Incline dumbbell fly - 1x20, 1x15, 1x12 reps

3. Machine chest fly - 1x20, 1x15, 1x12 reps

Quadriceps

1. Hack squats - 1x20, 1x15, 1x12 reps

2. Leg extensions - 1x20, 1x15, 1x12 reps

3. Holding dumbbell squats - 1x20, 1x15, 1x12 reps

4. Side lunges on bosu - 1x15, 1x15, 1x15 for each side

Tuesday

Shoulders

1. Side laterals - 1x20, 1x15, 1x12 reps

2. Front laterals - 1x20, 1x15, 1x12 reps

3. Rear laterals - 1x20, 1x15, 1x12 reps

Triceps

1. Triceps dip machine - 1x20, 1x15, 1x12 reps

2. Rope overhead triceps extensions - 1x20, 1x15 reps

3. W-bar skull crushers - 1x20, 1x15 reps

Thursday

Back

1. Under grip pull downs - 1x20, 1x15, 1x12 reps

2. Pull down to front - 1x20, 1x15, 1x12 reps

3. T-bar rows - 1x20, 1x15, 1x12 reps

4. Seated back pulley rows - 1x20, 1x15, 1x12 reps

Hamstrings

1. Dumbbell deadlifts - 1x20, 1x15, 1x12 reps

2. Supine hamstring ball curls - 1x15, 1x15, 1x15 reps

Calves

1. Plate loader calf pushes - 1x20, 1x15, 1x12 reps

2. Seated calf raises - 1x20, 1x15, 1x12 reps

Friday

Traps

1. Dumbbell shrugs - 1x20, 1x15, 1x12 reps

Biceps

1. Overhead cable curls - 1x20, 1x15, 1x10 reps

2. Bar pulley curls - 1x20, 1x15, 1x10 reps

Forearms

1. Cross the bench bar flexor curls - 1x20, 1x15 reps

2. Reverse barbell curls - 1x20, 1x15 reps

Core

1. Same workout as Sunday

EIGHT WEEK STRENGTH TRAINING PROGRAM FOR WOMEN

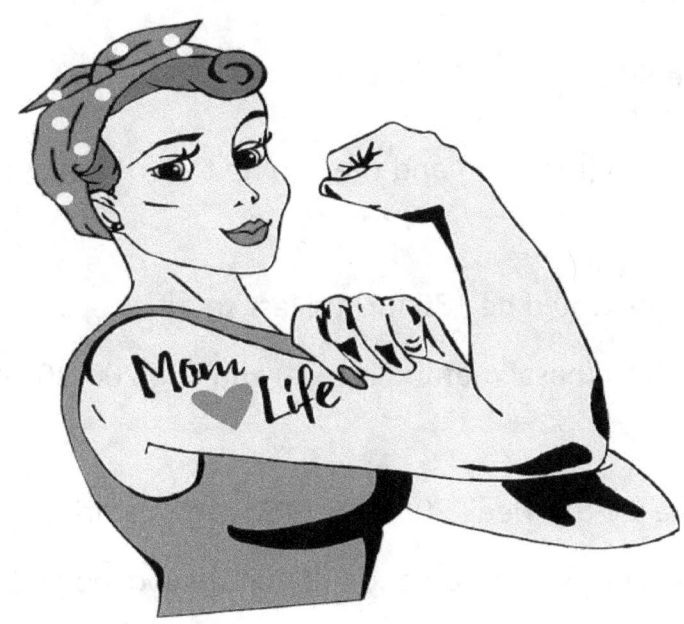

If you have completed the two week warm up program, you are now ready for the eight week training program.

If you are not a beginner, then jump right into this program. If you are not a beginner, just jump into this training program. If your level 2, add an extra set to each exercise to suit your needs.

Remember, if the volume of sets and repetitions are too much, then just reduce the amount to suit your individual needs.

Get ready to train and build some muscle!

8 Week Strength & Mass Building Program For Women – Level 1

Week 1: Heavy week

1. Figure out your 1RM (rep max) and then go up to 90% of your 1RM on your last set.

- a 200 lb bench press would be 180 for the last set of 4 reps

2. Figure out your BMR (basal metabolic rate) and add 200-300 calories extra per day.

- total caloric intake for the week 200 x7 = 1400 extra calories

3. Always do a 5-8 minute warm-up and 5-8 minute cool down before and after every training session.

This should include static stretching after each exercise session.

4. Use ascending pyramiding for all set and exercises throughout this program.

5. If you are unsure of any exercise just look it up on the internet.

6. Go to failure on the last set and record all your weights.

7. Rest 30-40 seconds in between on all sets and reps.

Sunday: Cardio 25-30 minutes + core

Monday: Back + hamstrings

Tuesday: Chest + triceps

Wednesday: Rest day

Thursday: Shoulders + biceps + core

Friday: Quadriceps + calves

Saturday: Rest day or light walking

Sunday

Cardio

1. Bike or tread mile – 25-30 minutes

Core

1. Hold Superman – 1x15, 1x15 seconds

2. Scissor kicks – 1x15, 1x15, 1x15 reps

3. Dumbbell crunches – 1x15, 1x15, 1x15 reps

4. Side planks – 1x15, 1x15 seconds each side

Monday

Back

1. Deadlifts - 1x10, 1x8, 1x6 reps

2. Reverse grip pull downs - 1x10, 1x8 reps

3. Barbell back rows - 1x10, 1x8, 1x6 reps

4. Lat pull down to front - 1x10, 1x8, 1x6 reps

Hamstrings

1. Lying leg curls - 1x10, 1x8, 1x6reps

2. Stiff legged dead lifts - 1x10, 1x8, 1x6 reps

Tuesday

Chest

1. Flat bench press - 1x10, 1x8, 1x6 reps

2. Dumbbell pullovers - 1x10, 1x8, 1x6 reps

3. Incline dumbbell fly - 1x10, 1x8, 1x6 reps

Triceps

1. Bar pulley push downs - 1x10, 1x8, 1x6 reps

2. Pulley rope overhead extensions - 1x10, 1x8reps

3. W-bar skull crushers - 1x10, 1x8 reps

Thursday

Shoulders

1. Seated barbell front press - 1x10, 1x8, 1x6 reps

2. Dumbbell side laterals - 1x10, 1x8, 1x6 reps

3. Bent over dumbbell rear laterals - 1x10, 1x8, 1x6 reps

Biceps

1. Barbell biceps curls - 1x10, 1x8, 1x6 reps

2. Seated machine biceps curls - 1x10, 1x8, 1x6 reps

Core

1. Same core as Sunday workout

Friday

Quadriceps

1. Plate loader leg press - 1x10, 1x8, 1x6, reps

2. Back squats - 1x10, 1x8, 1x6 reps

3. Leg extensions - 1x10, 1x8, 1x6 reps

4. Hack squats - 1x10, 1x8, 1x6 reps

Calves

1. Seated calf raises - 1x12, 1x10, 1x8 reps

2. Standing calf raises - 1x12, 1x10, 1x8 reps

Week 2: Medium- Light Week

1. Go up to 70% 1RM

- a 200 lb bench press would be 140 for 8 reps on the last set

2. Do not go to failure on any set

Sunday: Cardio 25-30 minutes + core

Monday: Chest + back

Tuesday: Shoulders + hamstrings + core

Wednesday: Rest

Thursday: Quadriceps + adductors + abductors + glutes + calves

Friday: Triceps + biceps + cardio

Sat: Rest

Sunday

Cardio

1. Tread mile or elliptical - 20-25 minutes

Core

1. Back extensions on the mat – 1x15, 1x15 reps

2. Reverse crunches – 1x15, 1x15, 1x15 reps

3. Cable crunches – 1x15, 1x15, 1x15 reps

4. Dumbbell side tilts - 1x15 each side

Monday

Chest

1. Regular or knee push ups - 1x15, 1x15, 1x15 reps

2. Incline dumbbell chest press - 1x15, 1x12, 1x10 reps

3. Cable crossovers - 1x15, 1x12, 1x10 reps

Back

1. Seated machine back row - 1x15, 1x12, 1x10 reps

2. Close grip pull down - 1x15, 1x12, 1x10 reps

3. One arm dumbbell back rows - 1x15, 1x12, 1x10 reps

4. High pulley pullovers - 1x15, 1x12, 1x10 reps

Tuesday

Shoulders

1. Machine shoulder press - 1x15, 1x12, 1x10 reps

2. Barbell upright rows - 1x15, 1x12, 1x10, 1x8 reps

3. Pulley face pulls - 1x15, 1x12, 1x10 reps

Hamstrings

1. Seated hamstring curls - 1x15, 1x12, 1x10 reps

2. Dumbbell dead lifts - 1x15, 1x12, 1x10 reps

Thursday

Quadriceps/adductors/abductors

1. Leg extensions - 1x15, 1x12, 1x10, 1x4 reps

2. Plie dumbbell squats - 1x15, 1x12, 1x10, 1x8 reps

3. Seated adductor machine - 1x15, 1x12, 1x10 reps

4. Seated abductor machine - 1x15, 1x12, 1x10 reps

Glutes

1. Table top glute kickbacks – 1x15, 1x15, 1x15 each leg

Calves

1. One legged standing dumbbell calf raises - 1x15, 1x12, 1x10 for each side

2. Seated calf raises - 1x15, 1x12, 1x10 reps

Core

1. Same core as Sunday

Friday

Triceps

1. Close grip bench presses - 1x15, 1x12, 1x10 reps

2. One arm overhead dumbbell triceps extension - 1x15, 1x12 each side

3. One arm dumbbell triceps kickbacks - 1x15, 1x12 each side

Biceps

1. Alternate dumbbell bicep curls - 1x15, 1x12, 10 reps

2. Preacher curls - 1x15, 1x12, 1x10 reps

Cardio

1. Treadmill or elliptical – 25-30 minutes

Week 3: Heavy Week

1. Go up 2.5-10lbs from week 1 on all exercises

2. A 2.5-5 lb increase on smaller muscle groups and a 5-10 lb increase on larger muscle groups

3. Go to failure on the last set

Sunday: Cardio 25-30 minutes + core

Monday: Back + hamstrings

Tuesday: Chest + triceps

Wed: Rest

Thursday: Shoulders + biceps + core

Friday: Quadriceps + calves

Saturday: Rest or light walking

Sunday

Cardio

1. Tread mile or rowing machine – 25-30 minutes

Core

1. Single prone leg lifts - 1x15, 1x15 reps

2. Bicycles - 1x15, 1x15, 1x15reps

3. Side plank reaches - 1x10, 1x10 each side

Monday

Back

1. Barbell back rows - 1x12, 1x10, 1x8 reps

2. Reverse grip pull downs - 1x12, 1x10, 1x8 reps

3. Bar deadlifts - 1x12, 1x10, 1x8 reps

4. Chin ups - 1x12, 1x10, 1x8 reps (use assisted chin up machine if necessary)

Hamstrings

1. Lying leg curls - 1x12, 1x10, 1x8 reps

2. Seated leg curls - 1x12, 1x10, 1x8reps

Tuesday

Chest

1. Flat bench press - 1x12, 1x10, 1x8 reps

2. Incline bench press - 1x12, 1x10, 1x8 reps

3. Incline dumbbell fly - 1x12, 1x10, 1x8 reps

4. Dumbbell pullovers - 1x12, 1x10, 1x8 reps

Triceps

1. Bar skull crushers - 1x12, 1x10, 1x8 reps

2. Pulley push downs - 1x12, 1x10, 1x8 reps

3. Pulley rope triceps overhead extensions - 1x12, 1x10, 1x8 reps

Thursday

Shoulders

1. Dumbbell side laterals - 1x12, 1x10, 1x8 reps

2. Seated barbell front shoulder press - 1x12, 1x10, 1x8, 1x6 reps

3. Bent over dumbbell rear laterals raises- 1x12, 1x10, 1x8 reps

Biceps

1. Seated machine biceps curls - 1x12, 1x10, 1x8 reps

2. Barbell biceps curls - 1x12, 1x10, 1x8 reps

Core

1. Same workout as Sunday

Friday

Quadriceps

1. Back squats - 1x12, 1x10, 1x8 reps

2. Leg press - 1x12, 1x10, 1x8 reps

3. Leg extensions - 1x12, 1x10, 1x8 reps

4. Hack squats - 1x12, 1x10, 1x8 reps

Calves

1. Standing calf raises - 1x12, 1x10, 1x8 reps

2. Seated calf raises - 1x12, 1x10, 1x8 reps

Week 4: Medium - Light week

1. Keep the same weights as week 2

2. We are increasing the resistance by increasing the reps

3. Do not go to failure for any sets

Sunday: Cardio 25-30 minutes + core

Monday: Chest + back

Tuesday: Shoulders + glutes + hamstrings

Wednesday: Rest

Thursday: Quadriceps + calves + core

Friday: Triceps + biceps + cardio

Saturday: Rest

Sunday

Cardio

1. Treadmill or elliptical – 25-30 minutes

Core

1. Bird dogs - 1x15, 1x15 reps

2. Dumbbell side tilts - 1x15, 1x15 each side

3. Stability ball passes - 1x12, 1x12, 1x12 reps

Monday

Back

1. Close grip V-bar pull down - 1x20, 1x15, 1x12 reps

2. Machine back row - 1x20, 1x15, 1x12 reps

3. High pulley pullovers - 1x20, 1x15, 1x12 reps

4. One arm dumbbell rows - 1x20, 1x15, 1x12 reps

Chest

1. Incline dumbbell chest press - 1x20, 1x15, 1x12 reps

2. Regular pushups - 1x20, 1x20, 1x20 reps

3. Cable crossovers - 1x20, 1x15, 1x12 reps

Tuesday

Shoulders

1. Machine shoulder press - 1x20, 1x15, 1x12 reps

2. Pulley face pulls - 1x20, 1x15, 1x12 reps

3. Barbell upright rows - 1x20, 1x15, 1x12 reps

Glutes

1. Table top glute kicks – 1x15, 1x15, 1x15 reps

Hamstrings

1. Dumbbell stiff legged dead lifts - 1x20, 1x15, 1x12 reps

2. Seated hamstring curls - 1x20, 1x15, 1x12 reps

Thursday

Quadriceps

1. Leg extensions - 1x20, 1x15, 1x12, 1x10 reps

2. Seated adductor machine - 1x20, 1x15, 1x12, 1x10 reps

3. Seated abductor machine - 1x20, 1x15, 1x12 reps

4. Plie dumbbell squats - 1x20, 1x15, 1x12, 1x10 reps

Calves

1. Seated calf raises - 1x20, 1x15, 1x12 reps

2. One legged standing dumbbell calf raises - 1x20, 1x15, 1x12 for each side

Core

1. Same workout as Sunday

Friday

Triceps

1. Seated overhead dumbbell triceps extensions - 1x20, 1x15, 1x12 reps

2. Close grip bench presses - 1x20, 1x15, reps

3. One arm dumbbell kickbacks - 1x20, 1x15 reps

Biceps

1. Preacher bar bicep curls - 1x20, 1x15, 1x10 reps

2. Alternate dumbbell biceps curls - 1x20, 1x15, 1x12 reps

Cardio

1. Bike or outside run – 25-30 minutes

Week 5 : Heavy Week

1. Figure out your 1RM

2. Go to up to 90% of your 1RM for all exercises.

3. Go to failure for the last set.

Sunday: Cardio 25-30 minutes + core

Monday: Chest + triceps

Tuesday: Back + biceps

Wednesday: Rest

Thursday: Chest/back (warm up) + Shoulders + core

Friday: Quadriceps + hamstrings + calves

Saturday: Rest or light walking

Sunday

Cardio

1. Elliptical or Rower – 25-30 minutes

Core

1. Hold superman – 1x20, 1x20 seconds

2. Dumbbell crunches – 1x20, 1x20, 1x20 reps

3. Scissor kicks – 1x20, 1x20, 1x20 reps

4. Side planks – 1x25 seconds each side

Monday

Chest

1. Flat dumbbell bench press - 1x10, 1x8,1x6 reps

2. Machine chest fly - 1x10, 1x8, 1x6 reps

3. Incline dumbbell bench press - 1x10, 1x8, 1x6 reps

Triceps

1. Rope triceps push downs - 1x10, 1x8, 1x6 reps

2. Decline dumbbell triceps extensions - 1x10, 1x8reps

3. Mini-dips - 1x12, 1x10 reps

Tuesday

Back

1. Close grip v-bar pull downs - 1x10, 1x8, 1x6 reps

2. Seated v-bar back pulley rows - 1x10, 1x8, 1x6 reps

3. Under grip chin ups - 1x10, 1x8, 1x6 reps (use assisted chin up machine if necessary)

4. One arm dumbbell back rows - 1x10, 1x8, 1x6 reps

Biceps

1. Machine biceps curls - 1x10, 1x8, 1x6 reps

2. Incline dumbbell biceps curls - 1x10, 1x8, 1x6 reps

Thursday

Chest/Back warm up (go lighter)

1. Machine pull down to front – 1x10, 1x8, 1x6 reps

2. Machine bench press – 1x10, 1x8, 1x6 reps

Shoulders

1. Seated dumbbell shoulder presses - 1x10, 1x8, 1x6 reps

2. Cable side laterals - 1x10, 1x8, 1x6 reps

3. Machine rear delt fly - 1x10, 1x8, 1x6 reps

Core

1. Same as Sunday

Friday

Quadriceps

1. Back squats - 1x10, 1x8, 1x6, 1x4 reps

2. Leg extensions - 1x10, 1x8, 1x6, 1x4 reps

3. Machine leg press - 1x10, 1x8, 1x6, 1x4 reps

Hamstrings

1. Standing leg curls - 1x10, 1x8 1x6 reps

2. Lying leg curls - 1x10, 1x8, 1x6 reps

Calves

1. Leg press machine calf pushes - 1x12, 1x10, 1x8 reps

2. Seated calf raises - 1x12, 1x10, 1x8 reps

Week 6: Medium Light Week

1. Go up 2.5-5 lbs for small muscle groups from week 4

2. Go up 5-10 lbs for larger muscle groups from week 4

3. Do not go to failure on any set

Sunday: Cardio 20-25 minutes + core

Monday: Chest + quadriceps

Tuesday: Shoulders + triceps

Wednesday: Rest

Thursday: Back + hamstrings + calves

Friday: Glutes + biceps + core +cardio

Saturday: Rest

Sunday

Cardio

1. Tread mile or bike – 25-30 minutes

Core

1. On stomach back extensions - 1x15, 1x15 reps

2. Cable crunches - 1x15, 1x15, 1x15 reps

3. Reverse crunches - 1x15, 1x15, 1x15 reps

4. Dumbbell side tilts - 1x15, 1x15 each side

Monday

Chest

1. Incline dumbbell flye - 1x15, 1x12, 1x10 reps

2. Flat machine bench press - 1x15, 1x12, 1x10 reps

3. Machine chest flye - 1x15, 1x12, 1x10 reps

Quadriceps

1. Holding dumbbell squats - 1x15, 1x12, 1x10, 1x8 reps

2. Leg extensions - 1x15, 1x12, 1x10, 1x8 reps

3. Side lunges on bosu - 1x15, 1x15, 1x15 for each side

Tuesday

Shoulders

1. Dumbbell front laterals - 1x15, 1x12, 1x10 reps

2. Dumbbell side laterals - 1x15, 1x12, 1x10 reps

3. Dumbbell rear laterals - 1x15, 1x12, 1x10 reps

Triceps

1. W-bar skull crushers - 1x15, 1x12, 1x10 reps

2. Rope pulley overhead triceps extensions - 1x15, 1x12 reps

3. Triceps dip machine - 1x15, 1x12 reps

Thursday

Back

1. T-bar rows - 1x15, 1x12, 1x10 reps

2. Seated back pulley rows - 1x15, 1x12, 1x10 reps

3. Under grip pull downs - 1x15, 1x12, 1x10 reps

Hamstrings

1. Supine one legged ball curls - 1x10, 1x10, 1x10 for each leg

2. Dumbbell stiff legged dead lifts - 1x15, 1x12, 1x10 reps

Calves

1. Seated calf raises - 1x15, 1x12, 1x10 reps

2. Plate loader leg press calf pushes - 1x15, 1x12, 1x10 reps

Friday

Glutes

1. Standing one legged pulley glute kicks – 1x15, 1x12, 1x10 each side

Biceps

1. Bar pulley biceps curls - 1x15, 1x12, 1x10 reps

2. Pulley overhead cable curls - 1x15, 1x12, 1x10 reps

Core

1. Same as Sunday workout

Cardio

1. Treadmill or bike – 25-20 minutes

Week 7: Heavy Week

1. Go up 2.5- 5lbs for smaller muscle groups from week 5

2. Go up 5-10 lbs for larger muscle groups from week 5

3. Go to failure for the last set

Sunday: Cardio + core

Monday: Chest + triceps

Tuesday: Back + biceps

Wednesday: Rest

Thursday: Chest/back (warm up) + shoulders + core

Friday: Quadriceps + hamstrings + calves

Saturday: Rest

Sunday

Cardio

1. Rower or Tread mile – 25-30 minutes

Core

1. Single prone leg lifts - 1x15, 1x15 each leg

2. Elbow plank – 30 seconds x 2

3. V-sit holds – 30 seconds x 2

4. Standing medicine ball twists - 1 minute x1

Monday

Chest

1. Incline dumbbell chest press - 1x12, 1x10, 1x8 reps

2. Machine chest fly - 1x12, 1x10, 1x8 reps

3. Flat dumbbell bench press - 1x12, 1x10, 1x8 reps

Triceps

1. Rope triceps push downs - 1x12, 1x10, 1x8 reps

2. Partial mini- dips - 1x12, 1x10 reps

3. Decline dumbbell triceps extensions - 1x12, 1x10 reps

Tuesday

Back

1. Close grip V-bar pull down - 1x12, 1x10, 1x8 reps

2. One arm back dumbbell rows - 1x12, 1x10, 1x8 reps

3. Under grip chin ups - 1x12, 1x10, 1x8 reps (use machine assisted chin ups if needed)

4. Seated V-bar back pulley rows - 1x12, 1x10, 1x8 reps

Biceps

1. Incline dumbbell curls - 1x12, 1x10, 1x8 reps

2. Machine biceps curls - 1x12, 1x10, 1x8 reps

Thursday

Chest/back (warm up)

1. Lat pull down to front – 1x12, 1x10, 1x8 reps

2. Machine bench press – 1x12, 1x10, 1x8 reps

Shoulders

1. Cable side laterals - 1x12, 1x10, 1x8 reps

2. Dumbbell shoulder presses - 1x12, 1x10, 1x8 reps

3. Machine rear delt fly - 1x12, 1x10, 1x8 reps

Core

1. Same workout as Sunday

Friday

Quadriceps

1. Machine leg press - 1x12, 1x10, 1x8, 1x6 reps

2. Leg extensions - 1x12, 1x10, 1x8, 1x6 reps

3. Back squats - 1x12, 1x10, 1x8, 1x6 reps

Hamstrings

1. Lying leg curls - 1x12, 1x10, 1x8 reps

2. Standing leg curls - 1x12, 1x10, 1x8 reps

Calves

1. Seated calf raises - 1x12, 1x10, 1x8 reps

2. Leg press calf pushes - 1x12, 1x10, 1x8 reps

Week 8: Light Medium Week

1. Use same weights as week 6 and we will increase resistance by reps

2. Do not go to failure any set

Sunday: Cardio + core

Monday: Chest + quadriceps

Tuesday: Shoulders + triceps

Wednesday: Rest

Thursday: Back + hamstrings + calves

Friday: Glutes + biceps + core + cardio

Saturday: Rest

Sunday

Cardio

1. Bike or tread mile – 25-30 minutes

Core

1. Land swimming – 1x20, 1x20 seconds

2. Stability ball pikes – 1x15, 1x15, 1x15 reps

3. Standing oblique bar twists - 1x1 minute

Monday

Chest

1. Flat machine bench press - 1x20, 1x15, 1x12 reps

2. Incline dumbbell fly - 1x20, 1x15, 1x12 reps

3. Machine chest fly- 1x20, 1x15, 1x12 reps

Quadriceps

1. Leg extensions - 1x20, 1x15, 1x12, 1x10 reps

2. Holding dumbbell squats - 1x20, 1x15, 1x12 reps

3. Side lunges on bosu - 1x15, 1x15, 1x15 for each side

Tuesday

Shoulders

1. Side laterals - 1x20, 1x15, 1x12 reps

2. Front laterals - 1x20, 1x15, 1x12 reps

3. Rear laterals - 1x20, 1x15, 1x12 reps

Triceps

1. Triceps dip machine - 1x20, 1x15, 1x12 reps

2. Rope overhead triceps extensions - 1x20, 1x15 reps

3. W-bar skull crushers - 1x20, 1x15 reps

Thursday

Back

1. Under grip pull downs - 1x20, 1x15, 1x12 reps

2. Pull down to front - 1x20, 1x15, 1x12 reps

3. T-bar rows - 1x20, 1x15, 1x12 reps

4. Seated back pulley rows - 1x20, 1x15, 1x12 reps

Hamstrings

1. Dumbbell deadlifts - 1x20, 1x15, 1x12 reps

2. Supine hamstring ball curls - 1x15, 1x15, 1x15 reps

Calves

1. Plate loader calf pushes - 1x20, 1x15, 1x12 reps

2. Seated calf raises - 1x20, 1x15, 1x12 reps

Friday

Glutes

1. Standing one legged pulley glute kicks – 1x20, 1x15, 1x10 each side

Biceps

1. Overhead cable curls - 1x20, 1x15, 1x10 reps

2. Bar pulley curls - 1x20, 1x15, 1x10 reps

Core

1. Same workout as Sunday

Cardio

1. Bike or elliptical – 25-30 minutes

CONCLUSION

Training. What does it mean? It doesn't mean running to the shoe store to get that special deal. In this book I have laid out the foundation for the process on how to get lean and how to gain muscle. It is up to you and consistency is key to achieving the best results. I have said this many times, you get what you put in. No one can put in 100% all the time. With family and work obligations, if you can give 80% to this process, you're doing good.

It is so easy to give up. Life throws challenges at you and it always will. Don't give up. Keep going and finish what you start. Only then will you get the physique you have always wanted.

MEET THE AUTHOR

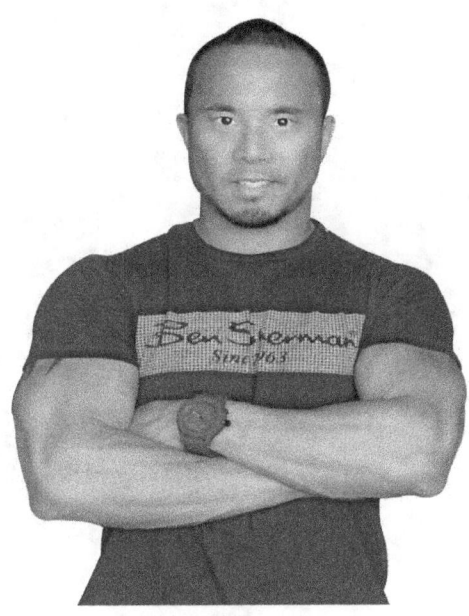

Paul Nam has been in the fitness industry and a personal trainer for over 20 years. He started bodybuilding at the age of 18 and became the Junior Mackenzie Bodybuilding Champion at 19. He has since then competed in over 25 bodybuilding, fitness, and martial arts competitions. He has trained in Olympic style boxing, Brazilian jui-jitsu, muay thai, wrestling, and holds a red belt in tae kwon do.

Paul owns a fitness studio in Toronto, builds mobile training apps, and is now writing a series of books. He also owns an online training business and builds fitness products.

Paul has been on numerous radio talk shows. He has also been a guest on the Nikki Clarke TV show and the Fitness Blitz podcast which reaches millions of people.

www.ingramcontent.com/pod-product-compliance
Lightning Source LLC
Chambersburg PA
CBHW081551280526
45788CB00011B/3432